the essentials in pressure monitoring

blood and other body fluids

DEDICATION

To my beloved wife Hanna and son, Mark, I dedicate this book.

Josef K. Cywinski.

THE TARDIEU SERIES

the essentials in pressure monitoring

blood and other body fluids

Jozef CYWINSKI, M.S.E.E., Ph.D., F.A.C.C.
Director of Medical Engineering Department, Massachusetts General Hospital Boston
Principal Associate in Anesthesia, Harvard Medical School, Boston Ma.
Lecturer, Harvard/MIT Health Science and Technology Program, Cambridge Ma.

and

Bernard TARDIEU
Medical Illustrator, Paris, France

Foreword by J. Warren HARTHORNE, M.D., F.A.C.C.
Associate Professor of Medicine, Harvard Medical School, Boston Ma.
Associate Physician, Massachusetts General Hospital, Boston Ma.

1980
MARTINUS NIJHOFF MEDICAL DIVISION - THE HAGUE
LONDON - BOSTON

Distributors :

for the United States and Canada

Kluwer Boston, Inc.
160 Old Derby Street
Hingham, MA 02043
USA

for all other countries

Kluwer Academic Publishers Group
Distribution Center
P.O. Box 322
3300 AH Dordrecht
The Netherlands

ISBN 90-247-2385-X (this volume)
ISBN 90-247-2352-3 (series)

PREFACE

''It's a small step for a man but a glant step for manking''. With these words Neil Armstrong capsulized the space age accomplishments of the sixties and seventies as he stepped onto the surface of the moon. While many achievements, both human and technical, contribued to he successful conclusion of this mission, a major contributing factor was provided by spectacular developments in the field of electronics. During subsequent years, a multitude of new devices founded upon improved electronic circuitry has made its way into our every day lives. Our children play casually with calculators and computer games, our automobile fuel injection systems are regulated by microprocessors and our hospitals have been re-equipped with sophisticated new diagnostic and therapeutic systems which scarcely existed a decade ago.

With regard to the latter application of this new electronic technology the underlying basic principles of patient monitoring have changed little despite the introduction of new, often intimidating appearing devices. It is to these principles that Dr. Cywinski directs this small text on patient monitoring. The eloquent illustrations by Mr. Bernard Tardieu further amplify these basic principles. The combination should create a substantial demand for this book by medical students, nurses, doctors in training practicing physicians and other paramedical personnel who may be thrust into the role of providing intensive monitoring of the seriously ill.

J. Warren Harthorne, M.D.
Associate Professor of Medicine
Harvard Medical School/Boston, Ma.

TABLE OF CONTENTS

FOREWORD

The direct pressure measurements and especially the blood pressures became routine method in intensive medical care. Blood pressure monitoring permits continuous assessment of cardiac performance, the volume of blood and status of blood vessels. The results of monitoring usually contribute to clinical diagnosis or its confirmation and to therapeutic interventions. The ability to monitor for long periods of time permits the assessment of the effectiveness of these interventions and often to their correction or change. Thus monitoring of pressures is an important factor in the quality of medical care and its outcome. While it affords faster recovery from life-threatening disease, there is as yet no quantitative measure of the degree to which it reduces mortality and morbidity. One qualitative logical conclusion can be stated: if and when properly used, blood pressure monitoring improves survival.

To be effective pressure monitoring has to be performed meticulously. Otherwise the complications and pitfalls will far outweigh the advantages. To learn proper technique for monitoring is not difficult—it simply requires effort and attention to detail.

It is easier to prevent mistakes than to cause them; hence the reason for this book. I have written it, aiming at the medical professionals in training—no scientists, engineers or administrators in health care.

This book provides practical, in-depth guidance to all who wish or have reason to use pressure monitoring in clinical practice.

I have deliberately excluded the complexity of medical and physical sciences underlying some principles involved in hemodynamic monitoring. This was done in order to keep the book transparently compact. My goal was to create a book to be used by those who wish to learn a practical skill or to teach others. The effectiveness and impact of the book will be judged by those who acquire such skill in pressure monitoring after using this modest volume.

This book would be nonexistant without help from all those I wish to thank for making it possible. First my friend, superb medical artist , illustrator of this book, constant inspiration, critic, editor, publisher and the moving force behind me Mr. Bernard Tardieu who indeed made this book into what it is. The medical review was brilliantly done by Warren J. Harthorne, M.D., a dear friend of mine and colleague. My pecial thanks also go to John Evans, M.D., for revising the first draft of the text and Mr. Franco Vitaliano whose editing talent in revising the chapter on historical review can only be surpassed by his own writing style which I consider the epitomy of word mastery. Ms. P. Carlson patiently edited, corrected and typed the manuscript and worked under pressure as well and devotedly as a partner would. Finally, to the staff of the Massachusetts General Hospital and to the Institution itself, whose contributions and support are too numerous to list here but which made this book a labor of love.

Jozef K. Cywinski, Ph.D.
Boston, March, 1980

I - BLOOD AND BLOOD PRESSURE: HISTORICAL REVIEW

The historical aspect of blood pressure is a fascinating subject. The earliest notions date back to the cavemen of Lascaux, who, 50,000 years ago, were apparently quite ware of the crucial importance to life of the heart and blood. In their striving to communicate this fundamental information, they painfully etched pictographs into their cave walls. No doubt, these images left a similarly deep impression upon their fellow tribesmen.

Indeed, everywhere in man's early writings are signs of his attempts to build a system of medicine and to describe the human anatomy. What I should like to do, then, is take you back through time and trace man's steps out of the dark caves of Lascaux towards scientific enlightenment.

From Lascaux, we travel forwards thousands of years, to 3000 B.C. We arrive on the great continent of Australia, and, as we listen to the chatterings of a primitive people around a campfire, we can hear the beginnings of legends that tell of, amazingly, successful blood transfusions. From Australia, we move to another great land mass, only a few hundred years later. It is now 2698 B.C. and we are in the court of the Emperor Hwang-Ti, ruler of ancient China. This man distinguished himself as being the first to produce scientific writings on cardiovascular circulation, and, what we are witnessing is the creation of one of the greatest, and most venerated of man's earliest medical textbooks: The Nei-Ching (Book of Medicine). Even though Hwang-wti's reign ended in 2599 B.C., this book is still studied and revered in contemporary China. While the exact publication date and true authorship still provide grist for the historian's mill, what is our care after we read these lyrical—yet oddly commanding lines: "The heart regulates all the blood in the body... the blood current flows continuously in a circle and never stops. The human body is like a chord instrument of which the different (pulsatile blood circulation-JKC) pulses are the chords... the harmony of discord of the organism can be recognized by examining the pulse, which is fundamental for all medicine. On it depends diagnosis, prognosis and therapy. Each pulse should be examined three times separately: first with light pressure, second with slightly more pressure, and thirdly with strong pressure... There are two hundred kinds of pulses; twenty-six of them may indicate approaching death..."[1].

It is clear from the above that pulse palpation and indirect blood pressure estimation were already a fundamental part of ancient Chinese medicine. From this set of exotic instructions it would appear that examination of a patient's pulse alone lasted several hours. The requisite skill, sensitivity, and patience of these early physicians had to be extraordinary.

But now let us prepare to travel forward again, this time 600 years and to the Middle East, the cradle of Western culture. We are in the Assyro-Babylonian kingdom, circa 2000 B.C. and some of history's earliest medical practitioners are starting to write what will become a medical textbook consisting of twenty-five thousand early cuneiform tablets. Eventually, they will become a part of the King Ashurbanipal's (668-626 B.C.) library at Ninive.

In this laboriously crafted text, a very important role was attributed to the blood as a magic carrier of every vital function. From these writings, Dawson[2] concludes that the liver was regarded as the seat of the essential life process. The liver was the organ into which all blood was received: hence, its importance.

Such was the growing recognition and fame for their pioneering efforts, that quite often, Assyrian and Babylonian physicians were called as far away as Egypt for consultations. Indeed, this is our next stop. Luxor, circa 2000-1800 B.C.; the peak of the twelfth dynasty's reign. According to Castiglioni[3], in the Ebers papyrus these early Egyptians wrote down that the cessation of respiration preceded the failure of blood circulation. Thus, they attributed the most important vital role to respiration. This pneumatic concept was a dominant characteristic in early Egyptian medicine. But not to be outdone was their equal regard for the importance of blood. Mummies were painted red to confer on them the strength of blood and amulets of reddish stones were placed around their necks for the same reason.These latter were symbols of the blood of the godess Isis.

As we stand in old Luxor, wer read in the Ebers, "The heart is the center of blood upply and there are vessels attached to it for every member of the body... the motion of the heart can be detected not only in the region of the heart itself but by placing the fingers on the head, the hands, the arms and the legs". Moreover, as we read on, we discover that they also knew the distribution and anatomy of the most important vessels.

These revolutionary ideas and their human recorders began finding their way onto ships that sailed down the great Nile, and then drifted out into the open seas, there to be seized upon by the early Greeks—Homer's contemporaries, who then set about expanding upon this precious cargo. First came the Pythagorean doctrine (580-489 B.C.) and the teachings of the Greek medical school of Croton. If we were to stop in around 500 B.C. we would hear Alcmaeon lecturing to his students that "Animal Life is a movement and subordinate to a movement of blood, which, if not always uniform, is continuous; that sensation and thought are subordinate to the invisible and unnoticed movement of the brain, and, that as movement is the essential factor to life, so diseases arise from a movement that disturbs the normal harmony of life"[3]. Later on, we would note Empedocles of Agrigentum (504-443 B.C.) stating that he believed respirations occurs ot only through the lungs, but also through the skin. "The blood is the carrier of heat acquired from respiration". And so that we should make no mistake in our priorities, he states that, "The heart is the first and most important organ formed in the fetus".

These and other teachings finally surfaced to produce the legendary Medical School of Cos, which in turn, gave us the father of scientific medicine: Hippocrates (459-355 B.C.). At the same time in the Far East the Chinese continued their interest in the circulation system as evidenced by a ten-volume treatise on the clinical appraisal of the arterial pulse published by Wang Chu Ho in A.D. 280.

But how far do we have to move forward from here? This time, our leap through space is herculean. We must rush past nearly two millenium before a mechanism of blood circulation is finally discovered. Only with this knowledge can the way be paved for the first quantitative estimates of blood pressure and circulation.

We are in London, and the year is now A.D. 1616. Sir William Harvey, educated in Padua, Italy, is quoting to us from his famous Lumleian Lecture: "The heart is an organ for the propulsion of blood and the valves in blood vessels are so arranged that the blood travels in one direction by going round and round. Encouraged by our attentiveness, he continues...". The blood in veins flows toward the heart and the valves placed at the beginning of the great arteries force the blood to move in precisely the opposite direction, away from the heart... the left side of the heart forces from itself at least two ounces of blood at each beat..." (Walker[4]).

Fifty-one years later, in 1667, we witness Denys performing the first scientifically recorded blood transfusions. Seven decades pass before we arrive at our next stop. Another Bristish scientist, and also clergyman, Rev. Stephen Hales, is transferring notes into his "Statistical Essays", a task that will take him from 1731 to 1733. We can see Reverend Hales busily writing down how he connected a glass tube into the femoral artery of a horse, and how, before his peers he directly measured the column of blood in the tube. He then demonstrated, to the amazement of his colleagues, that its height depended on the pressure within the artery. Not content to stop there, we observe him later on studying the benaviour of the pulse with his sphygmoscope, from which he managed to make good estimates of the cardiac output and blood velocity in mammals.

Now, things start happening quickly; the pivotal years flash past with hardly a chance for us to catch our breath.

We are in 1816, and another important chapter in the history of blood pressure measurement is being written as Laennec invents the medical stethoscope. A scant twelve years later, in 1828, Poiseuille invents the hemodynamometer. His invention was an adaptation of a mercury manometer to facilitate direct blood pressure measurement. Soon afterwards, in 1848, Ludwig, placing a mobile float with a writing point inside the hemodynamometer, *records* the first direct arterial mean pressure of a human, on a smoked drum kymograph. Poiseuille, not to be outdone by his confrere, goes on to invent a blood viscosimeter, and with it, he makes such progress in the study of blood that he derives mathematical equations quantitizing it now known as Poiseuille's law.

In 1855, Karl Von Vierordt is reporting the first non invasive sphygmograph, and in 1858, he goes on to invent a hemotachometer for recording blood velocity. Further inventions leading to our present state-of-the-art happen quickly. We observe Rica Rocci in 1896 developing the quantitative indirect blood pressure measurement method, with an airpressurized occlusive cuff. In 1904, Pachon is seen further developing this concept with oscillatory sensing of cessation of blood flow in a cuff-pressed radial artery. Then, one year later, Korotkoff develops an auscultatory method for non-invasive detection of systolic and diastolic blood pressures such as is used today (Bellvilee and Weavers[5]).

As we move towards 1912. Hurter is investigating the technique for puncturing a human radial artery for the twin purposes of blood pressure measurement and blood sampling. This technique is used by Stadie in 1919. In 1924, we watch Forssmann inserting a long catheter into his own antecubital vein and attempting to analyse the blood from his own right atrium. In 1934, Landis is seen measuring the blood capillary pressure with a micropipette. Suddenly, it is 1941, and Cournand has developed Forssmann's method further to permit graphic registration over considerable time intervals. If we watch him closely, monitoring the instruments, we can see how he establishes that the right atrial pressure ranges normally from 0 to 2 mmHg (millimeters of mercury), and that in cases of cor pulmonale, it may rise as high as 8 mm.

If we had been observant during the 20th century, we would have noticed the parallel developement of technologies to support these discoveries. In 1903, Frank could have been seen inventing the optical manometer, finally to be improved upon by Hamilton in 1934, when the metallic diaphragm was added. We might also have witnessed Lilly inventing the capacitance manometer in 1947, the forerunner of today's electronic pressure transducer.

And so, we arrive in the present. It would have been interesting to travel about some more, but the scope of this cahpter is unfortunately limited.

What do we see when look about ourselves today?

We very quickly become aware that since the early 1970's the equipement for direct blood pressure and cardiac function measurement has become so functional, reliable, and easy to use, that it now constitutes a mainstay of almost every intensive care facility. The vital importance of blood pressure has become evident even to the layman.

However, let us always bear in mind that it took some 50,000 years of human curiosity, imagination, risk-taking, and sheer effort for the following definitions to appear below, as reprinted from the 1977 ed. of Readers Digest Great Encyclopaedic Dictionary:

BLOOD: The fluid circulating through the vascular system of animals... that delivers oxygen and nutrients to the cells and tissues, distributes internal secretions, guards against infections and helps to maintain homeostasis of the organism.

BLOOD PRESSURE: The pressure of the blood on the walls of the blood vessels, varying with the force of the heart action, resilience of vessels, amount and viscosity of blood, etc.

BIBLIOGRAPHY

1. WONG-WU: "History of Chinese Medicine", *Tientsin,* 1932.
2. DAWSON, W.R.: "The Beginnings, Egypt and Assyria", *Hoeber, N.Y.* 1930
3. CASTIGLIONI, A.: "A History of Medicine", *2nd ed., A. Knopf, publ., N.Y.* 1947.
4. WALKER, K.: "The Story of Medicine", *Oxford Univ. Press, N.Y.,* 1955.
5. BELLVILLE, J.W. and WEAVER, Ch.S.: "Techniques in Clinical Physiology", *MacMillan Co., London,* 1969.

II - PHYSICS OF FLUID PRESSURES

2.1. Force and pressure

All material objects are attracted towards the earth by the *force of gravity*. This fact of course also applies to liquids. This *force of attraction* (meaning the force at the surface of our planet) is called the *weight* of the object and it is directly proprotional to its *mass*.

For example, a glass full of water has a larger mass than one filled with air, and it also has a proportionately greater weight. Similarly, a unit volume of whole blood weighs more than the same volume of saline. Both weigh much less than the same volume of mercury which is the heaviest (densest) liquid. The ratio of the amount of force (weight) to the surface area to which this force is applied is called *pressure*. The greater the force the greater the resulting pressure; also, the smaller the area the same force is applied to, the greater the resulting pressure. A glass of water standing on a table surface exerts more pressure than does the same glass filled with air. This is because water provides more weight (i.e. force) than the air to the *same* table surface area. An example illustrating the pressure relation to force and area is the case of two syringes of different volumes and of different diameters. Applying the *same* force to the piston of each syringe will result in a much *greater* pressure delivered by a smaller syringe (Fig. 1)

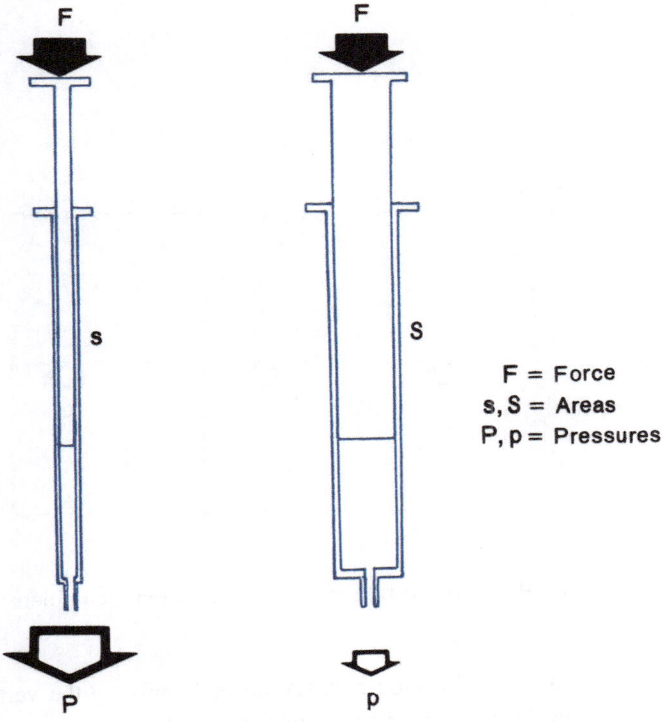

Fig. 1 - Two syringes produce different pressures even when the same force is used

2.2. Pressure in fluids

A fluid is a substance which can flow. Both gases and liquids fall into this category. The main difference between the two lies in their compressibility, i.e., the ease (force) with which their volume can be reduced. Gases are easily compressible while liquids are virtually not. Observing this fact of incompressibility, *Pascal* described a physical *Law* stating that a *change of pressure at any point in liquid results in a like change anywhere in the entire volume of the liquid.* This law has a significant meaning for the quantitative measurements of blood pressure.

Let us now imagine two glasses on the surface of the table. One glass is filled with water and the other is only half full. The resultant pressure on the surface of the table will be exactly half under the glass half full in respect to the full glass. Naturally, the pressure depends on the height of the fluid column exerting it. Furthermore, the pressure varies with this height in a linear fashion: *the higher the column, the higher the pressure*. This is an essential concept in the measurement or monitoring of blood and other fluid pressures. In addition, this so-called *hydrostatic pressure* does not depend on the shape or volume of the glasses in our example. It depends *only* on the *vertical height* of the column and *density* of fluid above the table surface. It is obvious that the same glass filled to the brim with mercury will exert 13·6 times greater pressure than the same glass filled with water, because mercury is 13·6 times denser than water (Fig. 2).

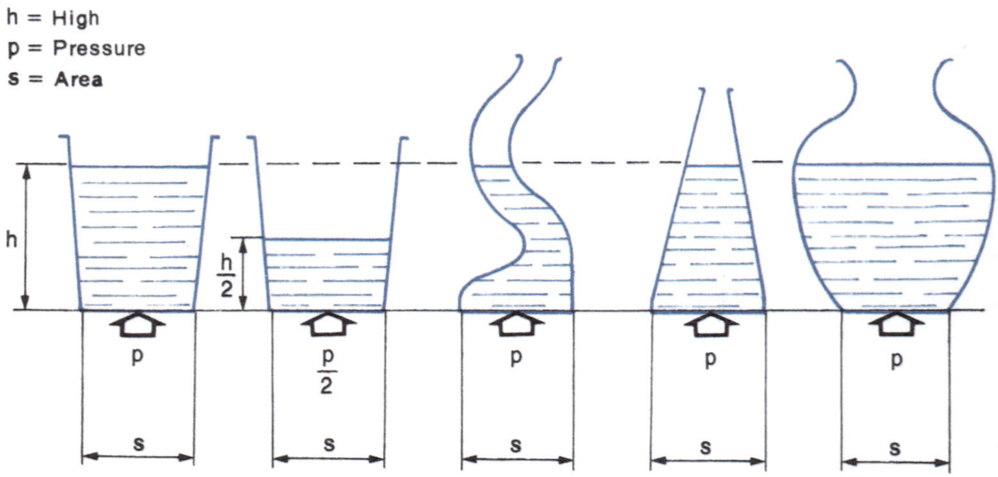

Fig. 2 - Pressure exerted by fluids in different containers

The fact that the hydrostatic pressure depends only on the vertical height of the column but no on the volume or shape of the vessel, seems at first glance puzzling. However, liquids which are incompressible and subject to Pascal's law, have an equal pressure distribution throughout their entire volumes.

2.3. Atmospheric pressure

The earth is surrounded by atmosphere which is a large volume of air. Air is attracted to the earth by the force of gravity. Therefore, the air of the atmosphere exerts a force on all objects exposed to it. This force exerted upon a unit area is called *atmospheric pressure*. Atmospheric pressure varies with altitude (because of the height of the air) and environmental conditions (climate) due to changes in air density. All clinical blood pressure measurement are made relative to atmospheric pressure.

2.4. Pressure measuring units

In the Bristish Unit convention system, the pressure is measured in *pounds per square inch* (psi). The atmospheric pressure at sea level equals 14·7 psi under normalised environmental conditions. In every day life (automobile type pressure) as well as in the industry of Northern America, psi units are widely used. In Europe and other countries where the metric system is used, pressures are measured in *Atmosphere* (Atm.). One Atm. corresponds to the pressure exerted by the force of one kilogram on a surface of 1 square meter.

In medicine, however, as in meteorology, a different units have been traditionally used for the quantitative expression of pressures : the *millimeter of mercury* (mmHg) or *centimeter of water* (cm H_2O). This looks like a paradox: pressure measured in units of length? The reason for this lies in the human tendency to describe physical phenomena with reference to the tools that happen to be available. The measurement of blood pressure was first accomplished (Hales, see p. 15) by observing the height of the column of blood rising in a tube inserted into an artery in a mare's neck. Later, tubes filled with mercury proved more compact and convenient (Poiseuilles, see p. 15). The height of mercury or water in the column was accepted as an indicator of pressure because the force of gravity is virtually constant on the earth's surface. The pressure unit based on and equal to mmHg is the *Torr*, to commemorate the Italian scientist Torricelli. Thus, 1 mmHg = Torr (on the earth's surface).

Now, during the era of space travel such units are losing their meaning. An International System (S.I.) of units has been adopted, where all the units are referred to either absolute standards or to physical laws deriving from these. Hence the new, modern unit for pressure is metric, and is defined as a force of 1 Newton per 1 square meter. These units are called *Pascals* to commemorate the famous physicist. For those who are not familiar with the name Newton as a unit of force, it is the force required to accelerate a mass of 1 kilogram at a rate of 1 meter per square second. Using these units there is no need to be on the earth's surface, at sea level, or to measure the height of the mercury column, in order to determine the pressure.

2.5. How to convert mmHg to cmH_2O to Pascals

In modern medical text, pressures are expressed in Pascals, and are sometimes given in parallel in mmHg or Torrs. It is useful then to know how to convert from one to the other.

The formula is: 1 mmHg = 133·3 Pascals (P) = 0·133 kilo Pascals (kP)

and in reverse: 1 Pascal (1 P) = 0·0075 mmHg

1 kilo Pascal (1kP) = 7·5 mmHg

The table below gives convenient values for conversion of pressure units within the common medical range. It also lists yet another linear (and traditionnaly oldest) pressure measure: the height in centimeters of a vertical column of water.

mmHg	cmH_2O	kP	kP	mmHg	cmH_2O	cmH_2O	mmHg	kP
0	0	0	0	0	0	0	0	0
1	1.36	0.133	0.1	0.75	1.02	1	0.735	0.0980
2	2.7	0.266	0.2	1.50	2.04	2	1.470	0.1960
3	4.1	0.399	0.3	2.25	3.06	3	2.205	0.2941
4	5.4	0.532	0.4	3.00	4.08	4	2.940	0.3922
5	6.8	0.655	0.5	3.75	5.10	5	3.675	0.4902
6	8.2	0.798	0.6	4.50	6.12	6	4.410	0.5882
7	9.5	0.931	0.7	5.25	7.14	7	5.145	0.6863
8	10.9	1.064	0.8	6.00	8.16	8	5.880	0.7843
9	12.2	1.197	0.9	6.75	9.18	9	6.615	0.8824
10	13.6	1.33	1.0	7.50	10.20	10	7.350	0.9804
20	27	2.66	2.0	15.00	20.40	20	14.700	1.960
30	41	3.99	3.0	22.50	30.60	30	22.051	2.941
40	54	5.32	4.0	30.00	40.80	40	29.40	3.922
50	68	6.55	5.0	37.50	51.00	50	36.75	4.902
60	82	7.98	6.0	45.00	61.20	60	44.10	5.882
70	95	9.31	7.0	52.50	71.40	70	51.45	6.863
80	109	10.64	8.0	60.00	81.60	80	58.80	7.843
90	122	11.97	9.0	67.50	91.80	90	66.15	8.824
100	135	13.33	10.0	75.00	102.00	100	73.50	9.804

Table I - Useful conversions for pressure measurement units

2.6. Pressure reference

Pressure does not exist in isolation. Pressure is a relationship of a difference in forces per unit area between two points. All medical measurements are *made with respect* to *atmospheric pressure,* which was arbitrarily established as *zero*. Hence all devices to measure or monitor medical pressures should read zero when exposed to atmosphere. Any given point in the blood circulatory system may have a different pressure when referred to the atmosphere with respect to another point within the same system.

2.7. Fluid flow resulting from pressure

If there is a zero pressure difference between two points, the fluid will not move. Whenever there is a pressure difference between two points in the fluid-filled system, the fluid will move in the direction of lower pressure to reach equilibrium. The movement of the fluid and the speed by which the pressure will equilibrate depends on the presence or absence or physical obstructions on the fluid pathway. These obstructions will govern the fluid flow from the higher to lower pressure region. More detailed discussion of this every subject in relation to blood pressures in the circulatory system will be presented in the next chapter.

III - BLOOD PRESSURE AND PULSE

3.1. Why is blood pressure important?

Blood is life. For the patient in a hemorrhagic shock due to massive bleeding after injury, life or death depends on the *maintenance* of *adequate blood pressure* and blood supply to the brain.

Blood must flow in order to supply vital oxygen and nutrients to organs and tissues. The pumping action of the heart results in pressure (force per unit area) causing the blood to flow from the heart to the arteries. Obstructions of the blood flow to vital organs may severely limit their functions. When the blood flow in a certain artery is completely obstructed (e.g., by a blood clot or thrombus), the issue in the area supplied by this vessel will die. Such an obstruction in a brain artery is one of the causes of stroke. An obstruction of a coronary artery which supplies blood to the heart may cause myocardial infarction. A blood clot in the lungs (embolism) may cause infarction of lung tissue. Most of these events have severe, and often fatal, results.

It is of *great medical importance* to be able *to determine* those factors which govern blood flow and, specifically, the *blood pressure* in seriously ill persons.
The need for *blood pressure monitoring,* especially for patients in shock or with cardiovascular problems, becomes critical.

3.2. What is blood pressure?

The commonly used term "blood pressure" means blood pressure in the arteries. The pressure is equivalent to the lateral force exerted by the blood per unit area of the arterial wall. The pressure in the circulatory system is the result of heart contraction force exerted on the blood in the ventricles. It is then ejected from the heart into the arteries. They have the capability of altering their cross sectional surface area by constriction or dilatation. Hence the blood pressure depends on both the heart force and cross sectional area of the arteries. This is true only in gross terms, because in reality the pressure and the mechanical properties of arteries are dynamically and rapidly changing, so that Pascal's laws governing pressures in liquids are severely limited. To get some understanding of the factors ruling blood pressure, a review of some facts from the field termed "hemodynamics" is useful.

3.3. Some hemodynamic terms

The arterial blood pressure is constantly pulsating with the pumping action of the heart. The latter contracts rhythmically approximately 70 times per minute, each of the contractions constituting a single cardiac cycle. During each cycle, the heart muscle exerts a force on the blood with which it is filled. This results in an ejection of a quantity of blood into the arteries called: the *stroke volume*. The sum of the stroke volumes over a period of one minute is called *cardiac output*.

It is obvious that blood flows out of the heart in boluses, hence the force causing this blood to flow is also pulsating as the heart muscle changes its contractile state during each cycle. From the physical definition (see Ch. 2), relating pressure to force, it follows that arterial blood pressure is also constantly changing during the course of a cardiac cycle. The highest arterial pressure almost corresponds to the moment when the heart muscle is in its strongest contraction: this is called *systolic pressure*.

The lowest pressure in the arteries occurs when the heart is in its maximally relaxed state: this is *diastolic pressure*.

A typical blood pressure is usually expressed as two slashed numbers; the *first* denotes systolic, and the *second,* diastolic arterial pressure. For example, a record of 120/80 mmHg means that systolic pressure is 120 and diastolic is 80 mmHg. The *arithmetic difference* between the two pressures is called the *pulse pressure*.

3.3.1. Mean pressure

Somewhere between systolic and diastolic pressure values, lies *mean pressure*. It is an average pressure which would have existed if all peaks of systolic pressure had been levelled with all valleys of diastolic pressure. (Fig. 3).

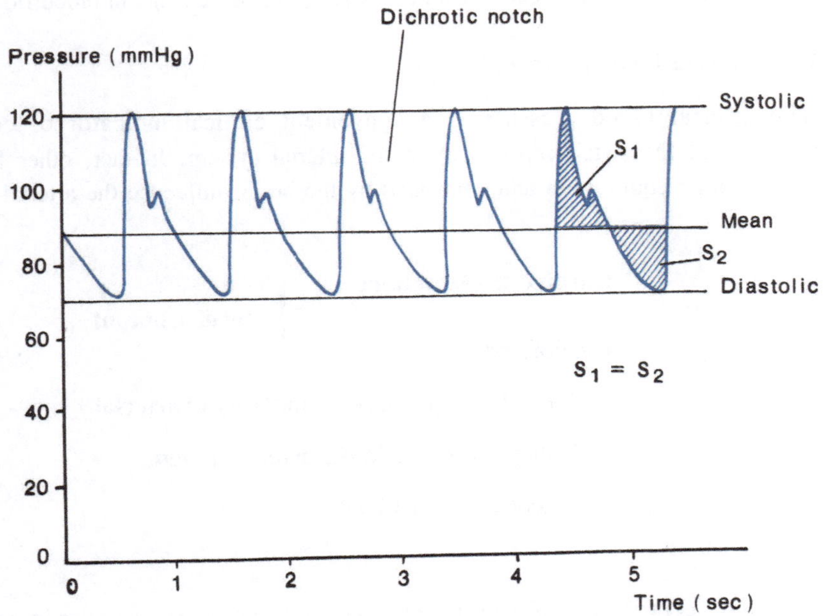

Fig. 3 - The components of arterial pressure and deviation of mean pressure

In clinical situations, mean pressure is a very useful value. It is usually determined by electronic or mechanical devices which perform this peak-and-valley levelling operation automatically on all momentary (instantaneous) pressure values over a period of time (several seconds). Such devices are called *time-averagers* or integrators. However, one can estimate the approximate mean pressure value for each cardiac cycle by the formulae:

$$\textbf{Mean pressure} = \textbf{Diastolic} + \textbf{1/3 pulse pressure or} = \frac{\textbf{systolic} + (\textbf{2} \times \textbf{diastolic})}{\textbf{3}}$$

As the true mean pressure is the time-average of the instantaneous presssure, the above formulae are highly inaccurate. Bruner[1] states that these formulae have substantial limitations and are useless for patients under the influence of vasopressor drugs or anesthesia.

3.3.2. Vascular impedance

Blood pressure within a given segment of the artery, and the amount of blood which flows through it, are interrelated. It is a commonsense notion that *the higher the pressure, the greater the blood flow*. Yet, there is still another factor to be taken into account: *vascular resistance*, or more generally, *vascular impedance*. The term "impedance" implies a factor of opposition to change. In the case of arterial blood pressure and flow, it is the ratio of the change in pressure to the change in flow. High impedance, (the radio of pressure to flow is high), for example, means that a large change in pressure will be associated with a relatively modest change in blood flow.

3.4. What governs blood pressure?

The arterial blood pressure is a convenient clinical indicator of cardiac performance and the state (impedance) or the arterial system. In fact, other factors acting in dynamic equilibrium and controlled by the brain, influence the arterial blood pressure:

Cardiac stroke volume } **cardiac output**
Cardiac rate }

— Vascular impedance & elasticity of arterial

— Volume of blood in the arterial system

— Viscosity of the blood

The exact contribution of each factor is not fully know but vascular impedance and cardiac output have definitely the greatest influence on arterial blood pressure.

3.5. Cardiovascular system structure

To clarify the behavior of the pressure pulse throughout our organism, let us first briefly review the structure of the cardiovascular system (Pl. 1, p. 50).

Oxygenated blood flows from the left ventricle of the heart into the systemic arteries characterized by a relatively high mean pressure of approximately 100 mmHg. The *arteries* branch into *arterioles* in which mean pressure drops to 40-25 mmHg. In their turn, arterioles branch into *capillaries* with mean blood pressure of 25-12 mm Hg. It is in the capillaries that the exchange of nutrients, oxygen, waste and carbon dioxide from the tissues takes place. The capillaries in turn converge into *venules* (12-8 mmHg) and *terminal veins* (less than 8 mmHg). The veins converge into the *vena cava* which returns the blood carrying waste products and CO_2 to the right atrium at a pressure of 3-2 mm Hg. The heart pumps the blood out from its right ventricle into lungs, where carbon dioxide is replaced by fresh oxygen. Oxygenated blood then flow into the left atrium and left ventricule where the systemic circulation originates. Thus, the blood completes two consecutive circulatory circuits: left ventricule to right atrium via systemic circulation, and right ventricle to left atrium via pulmonary circulation.

As outlined above, both the mean pressure and total flow are highest in the aorta, where the blood leaves the heart. Blood flow is a function of the blood pressure and of the impedance of the vessels. Both the impedance and the blood pressure in the capillaries and arterioles can vary over a wide range. For instance, when exposed to low temperatures or certain drugs (e.g., nicotine), the body reduces the blood flow through the skin by *vasoconstriction* (narrowing) of the arterioles. Heat, excitement, drugs or local inflammation cause *vasodilatation* (widening) of the arterioles, which locally, increases the blood flow. Fruthermore, the vascular impedance of the arteries increases with their distance from the heart. This is due to the geometry (size) of the vessels and mechanical properties of their walls.

3.6. The pressure pulse

What we commonly know and understand as a *peripherial pulse* is in fact a *pressure pulse*. It is important to assess the impact of the pressure pulse characteristics on the indices of blood pressure as measured in medical practice.

The pressure pulse varies according to where and how it is observed. In general, the pressure pulse travels from the left ventricle to the periphery, the right heart, the pulmonary circuit, and back to the left heart atrium. It has been shown that the pressure pulse travels faster than blood flow. Its velocity, according to Milnor[3] in the range 3 to 14 meters per second, which is 15 to 100 times the rate of blood flow. Furthermore, this *velocity* depends on the rate-of-change of the pressure. This fact, combined with variability of vascular impedance, is responsible for the changes in the pressure pulse as it travels through the aorta, arteries, arterioles, etc. The branching of the arterial tree results in an increase in arterial impedance. This causes a progressive rise in the peak systolic value of the pressure pulse as it travels further away from the heart. The complexity of the situation is enhanced by the reflection of the pressure pulse at the termination of peripheral arterioles setting up resonance in the arterial system. This results in further increase of the peak systolic value, and narrowing of the entire pressure pulse waveform.
(Fig. 5).

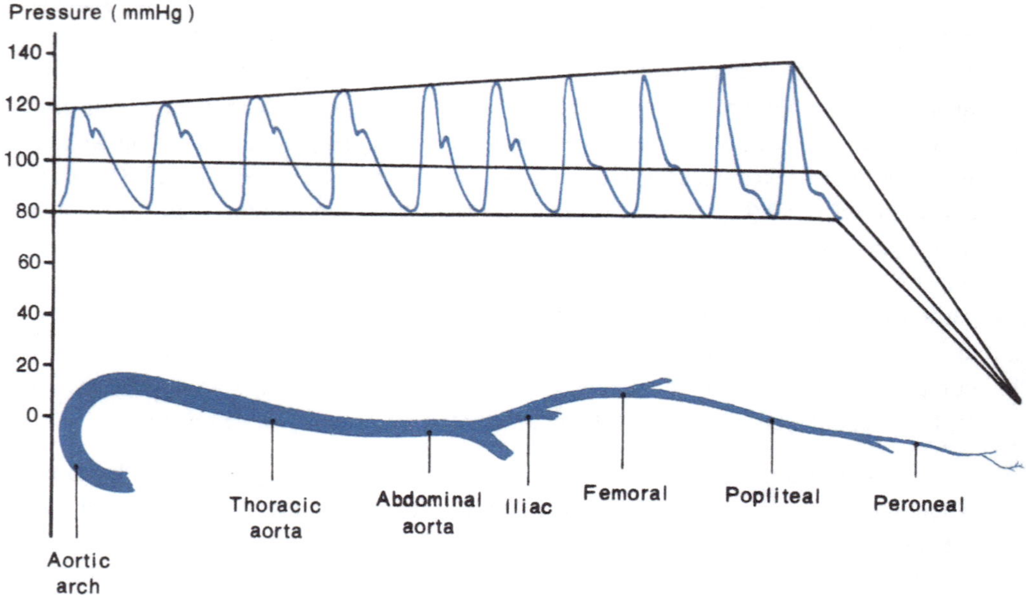

Fig. 4 - Differences in pulse pressure at several sites in the arterial system

In effect then, the pressure pulse in the peripheral artery may be markedly different from the one observed closer to the heart. The major difference is the shortening of systole and heightening of the systolic pressure the further away from the heart it is measured. Bruner[1] pointedly states that: "drugs, respiration and global changes in the circulation markedly affect the caracter of the pressure pulse... It is appropiate, though, to regard with enlightened skepticism the perceived numbers and waves, and to be both cautious and humble in drawing conclusions and in manufacturing presumptively therapeutic interventions."

BIBLIOGRAPHY

1. BRUNER, J.M.R., "Handbook of Blood Pressure Monitoring", *PSG Publ. Co., Littleton, Ma.* 1978.
2. CYWINSKI, J.K., "Direct Monitoring of Blood Pressure", *Bell and Howels, Pasadena, Ca.* 1977.
3. MILNOR, W.R., "Pulsatile blood flow", in Physiology in Medicine, *N. Engl. Jo. Med.*, **287:27,** 1972.

IV - INDIRECT MEASUREMENT OF BLOOD PRESSURE

4.1. Sphygmomanometry

The word "indirect" indicates that there is no direct physical contact between the manometer (pressure measuring device) and the source of pressure (i.e. blood vessel). There are several different methods available for indirect blood pressure measurement. The most popular indirect method is the use a *sphygmomanometer* with occlusive *cuff* placed over an arm and a *stethoscope*. The reader interested is the details of this method is referred to an AHA report on the subject 1,5.

4.1.1. The manometer, a vertical glass tube calibrated in millimeters (mm), connected to a reservoir containing mercury. The air-space above the mercury in the reservoir communicates with the compression bladder and with the pressure source via thick-walled flexible rubber tubes. The top of the vertical glass tube is vented to atmosphere. When there is no pressure difference, the mercury meniscus in the tube and the mercury level in the reservoir are identical. The mercury meniscus in the tube should be, in this case, at zero level. This corresponds to the situation when the cuff inflation bulb vave is open to air. When this valve is closed and pressure is exerted on the mercury in the reservoir, its level slightly falls, but the mercury in the glass tube rises. A given amount of pressure will always support a column of mercury of the same height in the upright tube. Once the mercury manometer is calibrated, recalibration is unnecessary. The *mercury manometers* is the *most reliable* and *simplest* instrument available for clinical measurements of blood pressure.

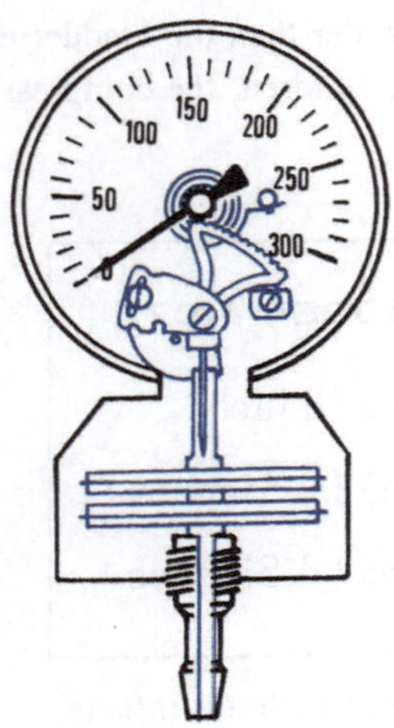

Aneroid manometer

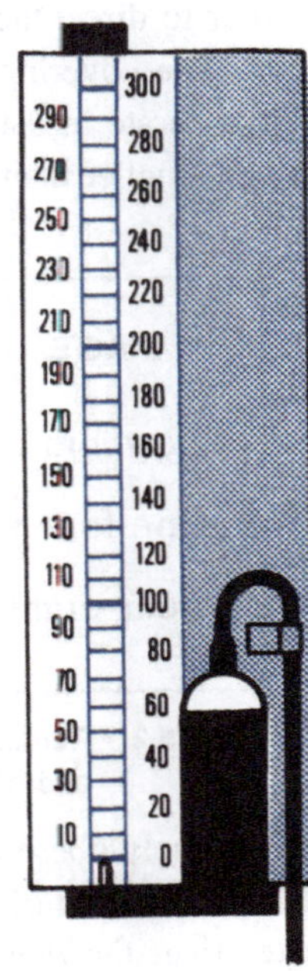

Mercury gravity type manometer

Fig. 5 - Manometers

For ease of portability, an *aneroid manometer* may be used instead of the mercury gravity type manometer (fig. 5). The aneroid consists of a metal bellows, the inside of which is connected to the compression cuff. Variation of the pressure inside the cuff causes the bellows to expand or collapse. This movement of the bellows rotates a gear that turns a needle across a calibrated dial.

Since the cuff pressure measured with the aneroid manometer depends on the elasticity of the metal bellows, it is subject to error. It is important to remember that the mere fact that the aneroid needle points to zero on the dial when the system is open to air, does not necessarily mean that the instrument is accurate within the entire pressure range. The aneroid manometer must be calibrated against a mercury manometer at regular intervals. A good, comprehensive discussion do sphygmomanometers and indirect blood pressure measurement was published by Baum[2,3].

4.1.2. The Compression Cuff, consisting of an inflatable rubber bladder within a non-elastic covering. The cuff is usually wrapped around the arm of the subject, in order o measure indirectly the blood pressure in the brachial artery. It has to be of the correct width according to the diameter of the patient's arm; if it is too narrow, the blood pressure reading will be erroenously high; if too wide, the reading will be erroneously low. The inflatable bladder should be long enough to encircle at least half of the arm diameter. The geometrical center of the bladder should be positioned over the artery being compressed. For the average-size adult arm, an inflatable bladder 13 cm. (5·1 inches) wide and 23 cm (9·1 inches) long, is usually satisfactory.

The covering which encloses and encircles the bladder is made of non-strech fabric in order to direct the compression exerted by the inflated bladder on the arm and not outward. The covering is one to two centimeters wider than the bladder and much longer. For accurate measurement of blood pressure in children, the compression cuffs must be much smaller than for adults. (Table 2).

AGE	BLADDER WIDTH
Newborn	2.5cm (1 inch)
One-four years	6 cm (2.3 inches)
Four-eight years	9 cm (3.5 inches)

Table 2 - Recommended widths of compression cuffs for infants and children

For extremely obese or slim patients, and also for measurement of blood pressure in legs, a correct width of the bladder must be selected. As a rule, this width must be 20% greater than the diameter of the limb on which it is used. The reason why an appropriate cuff width is necessary is to ensure that the compression pressure which is measured in the bladder, will be exerted on the artery over which it is positionned.

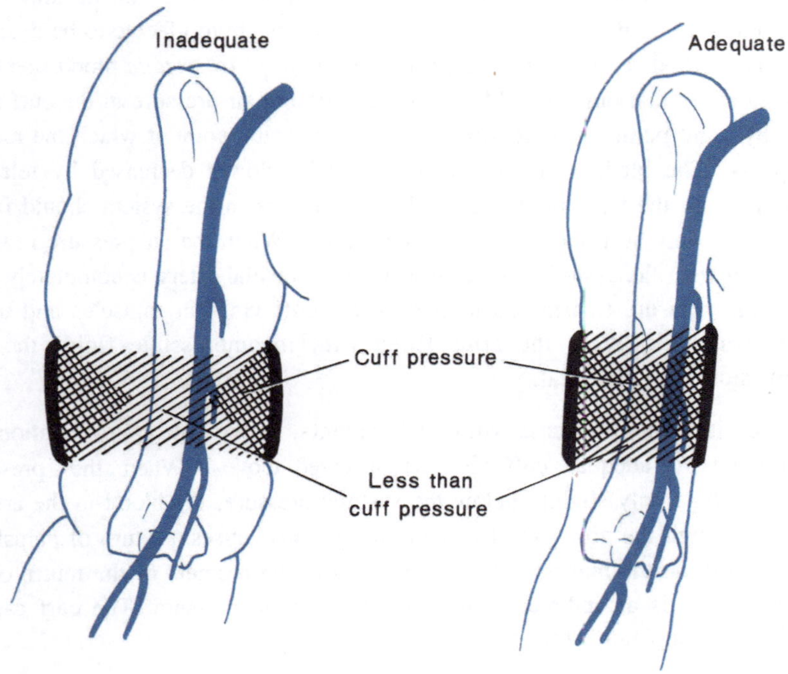

Fig. 6 - Cuff width influence on accurary of sphygmomanometer blood pressure reading

4.1.3. The pressure source, consisting of a rubber hand bulb pump and bleed control valve.

All the above recommendations as well as the following description of the method are bases on the American Heart Association's Commitee on Standardization of Blood Pressure Readings, published in *Jama*[5]. (Fig. 7).

4.2. The technique of blood pressure measurement using sphygmomanometers

The patient should be seated or lying down and well relaxed. The arm should be bared, slightly flexed, abducted and supported on a smooth surface.

The artery over which the blood pressure is to be recorded should be at the heart level. It is *not* necessary for a manometer to be at a level with the heart. Then the deflated cuff is wrapped evenly around the arm with the lower edge of the cuff about 1 inch above the antecubital space. If the veins of the arm are prominently filled, the cuff should be applied while the arm is elevated. The mercury column *must* be *vertical* and the meniscus should be read at a level with the observer's eye.

4.2.1. Palpation

It is advisable to take the sphygmomanometric blood pressure reading at least twice, each time using first palpatory, then the auscultatory method. In infants the latter often cannot be used because the auscultatory sounds are too feeble to be detected. The palpatory method serves as a preliminary measurement of *systolic* blood pressure *only*. The patient's radial pulse should be palpated and the air pressure in the cuff should be raised by hand pumping to approx. 30 mmHg over the point at which the radial pulse disappears. The bladder pressure then should be slowly decreased by releasing the bleed valve on the hand pump bulb. The air pressure in the system should fall slowly and continuously at a rate fo 2-3 mm per second. When the air pressure in the cuff is still higher than the systolic blood pressure, the brachial artery is completely collapsed due to the pressure transmitted to it from the cuff via skin, muscles and underlying tissue structures. Were the arms filled with incompressible fluid, the pressure transmission would be ideal.

Yet it is not the case with real patients, hence the approximation and the requirements for adequate cuff width as discussed above . When the pressure in the cuff falls only slightly below the systolic pressure, the blood in the artery starts flowing through the now partially open lumen. This causes a return of palpable pulse. The pressure on the manometer corresponding to the moment of the return of the first palpable pulse is an indirect estimate of the systolic pressure. The cuff can now be rapidly and completely deflated.

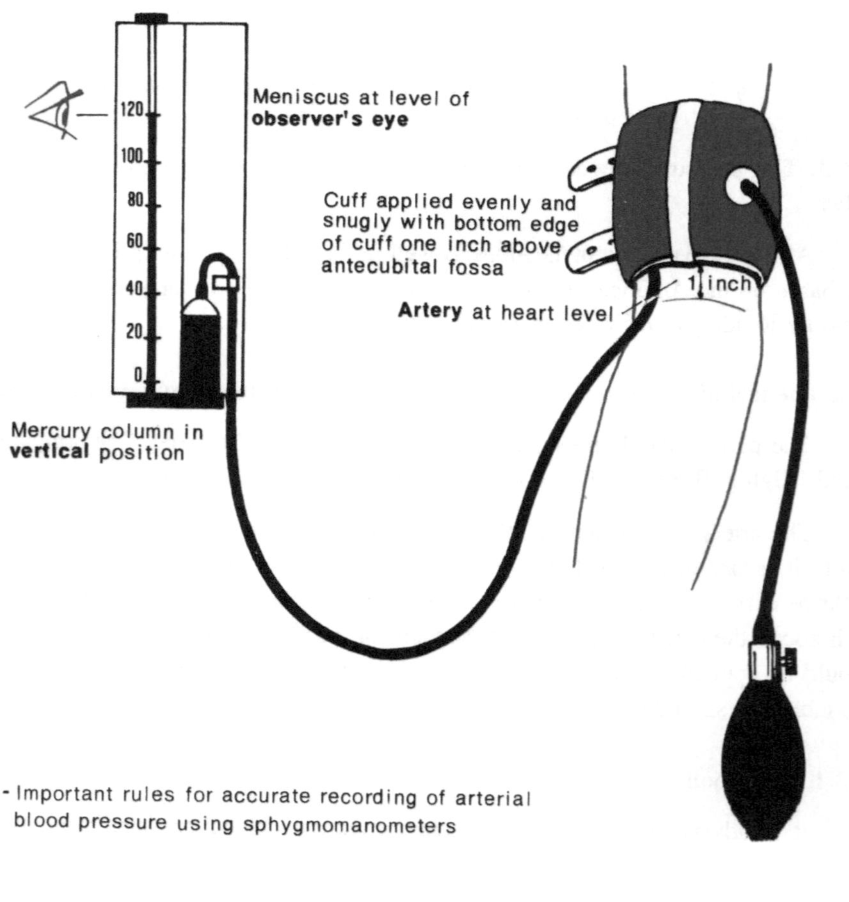

Fig. 7 - Important rules for accurate recording of arterial blood pressure using sphygmomanometers

4.2.2. Auscultation and Korotkoff sounds

The next determination of the arterial systolic and diastolic blood pressure will be performed using auscultatory method. With this method a stethoscope head should be applied to the antecubital space over the previously palpated brachial artery. The stethoscope should be applied with as little pressure as possible but with no air space between it and the skin. Heavy stethoscope pressure will distort the artery and produce an erroneous diastolic reading. With the stethoscope in place, the bladder is inflated using a hand bulb to a pressure approx. 30 mmHg higher than the point at which the radial pulse disappears. Then the bleed valve on the hand bulb should be slightly released to allow for slow and continuous deflation of the compression cuff. The rate of deflation should be 2-3 mmHg per second. Faster or slower deflation rates will result in erroneous reading of the pressure.

As long as the pressure in the cuff is higher than arterial pressure, the artery is completely compressed, and all sounds perceptible through stethoscope disappear. As the pressure falls, the so-called Korotkoff sounds become audible in the stethoscope placed over the artery below the cuff. At this moment, the artery is open for the blood to flow only during the peak of the pressure pulse, and is occluted during the remaining time of the pressure cycle. Thus, the arterial wall moves rapidly creating the sounds. It is worth emphasizing that Korotkoff sounds are due to the lateral movement (flapping) of the arterial walls, with their lumen partially opening and then completely closing during part of the pulse cycle. The Korotkoff sounds are not the heart sounds, but their rhythm is dictated by the heart contraction and ensuing pressure pulse. As the pressure in the cuff falls, the Korotkoff (''K'') sounds change character. There are five distinctive types of sounds, called *Phases,* each corresponding to a different cuff pressure level range.

- Phase I : ''K'' sounds occurs when the cuff pressure is slightly lower than systolic pressure. They first appear as faint, clear tapping sounds, which gradually increase in intensity. As the pressure falls, they are followed by:
- Phase II : the murmur or swishing quality sounds. As the cuff pressures continues falling, they are replaced by:
- Phase III : sounds which are crisper, and increase in intensity. As the pressure falls, there is.
- Phase IV : a distinct, abrupt muffling of noise, so that a soft, blowing sound is heard.
- Phase V : then, all sounds disappear.

At Phase V, the pressure in the cuff should be rapidly released. A few minutes should ellapse to facilitate the release of blood trapped in the veins, before any subsequent inflations of the cuff are made.

The muffling and disappearance of "K" sounds are commonly referred to as the fourth and fifth points.

The above description of sounds, as well as the following text is based on the American Heart Association's Recommendations for Human Blood Pressure Determination, published in Circulation, in 1967[5].

4.2.3. Blood pressure determination

● *Systolic pressure* is determined at the point at which the first tapping sound is heard for at last two consecutive beats. This corresponds to the beginning of Phase I. If and when the palpatory systolic pressure is higher it should be recorded and noted as systolic pressure.

● *Diastolic pressure* is the point when the muffling occurs at the end of Phase IV. The diastolic pressure estimated this way will be slightly higher (7-10 mm) than the actual diastolic pressure within the artery. The true equilibration of cuff and arterial pressure at the end of diastole occurs in Phase V and there are no audible sounds. There is difficulty for some observers in detecting the onset of phase V. If there is a different manometer reading of the fourth and fifth Phase (as frequently happens), both pressures should be recorded as follows : 142/82/78 mmHg where 82 corresponds to the 4th phase, 78 to the 5th. If the two levels are identical this should be recorded as : 142/78/78.

4.2.4. The effect of hydrostatic pressure: It is important to bear in mind to keep the forearm at heart level. When the patient is sitting upright, the compression cuff should be level with the fourth intercostal space. If the arm is raised the blood pressure reading will be too low, if lowered the reading too high. This effect is due to the hydrostatic pressure of the column of blood (see Chapter 2, of this publication). Disregard of this fact can cause errors in blood pressure readings as high as 10 mmHg. If the patient'arm cannot be positioned at the heart level during a blood pressure measurement, a correction for the hydrostatic pressure must be made. For each centimeter of vertical height above or below the heart level, 0·7 mmHg must be susbstracted or added, respectively, to the observed systolic and diastolic pressures.

4.3. Blood pressure measurement in the lower limb

For this measurement the patient should lie in the prone position. A cuff 20 to 22 cm wide (6 cm wider than the arm cuff) is usually adequate. The compression bladder is placed over the posterior surface of the midthigh. The stethoscope is positioned over the artery in the popliteal fossa, and the Korotkoff sounds are recorded as he cuff pressure is decreased in the same manner as in the arms. Accurate comparison of intra-arterial blood pressures in the arms and legs, in humans, shows that the femoral systolic pressure is only a few millimiters higher, and the diastolic one a few millimeters lower than brachial artery pressure. However, the pressures measured by indirect methods using 20 cm cuffs usually records systolic pressures 10-40 mm higher in the thigh than in the arms, altough diastolic pressures are essentially the same.

This systolic reading is clearly erroneous and is due to a poorer transmission of the pressure, from the compression cuff, through the structures inside the thigh, to the arterial walls.

There is a gradual dispersion of compression pressure on the way from the cuff to the artery; thus the cuff should be inflated above systolic pressure in order to stop the blood flow in the femoral artery.

4.4. Blood pressure reading in arrhythmias

Indirect blood pressure determination is highly inaccurate if the cardiac rhythm is very irregular. This is because stroke volume and left ventricular systolic blood pressure vary from one cardiac contraction to the next. A shortened cardiac contraction cycle results in increased diastolic and decreased systolic pressures. Conversely, a long cycle results in a reduction in the diastolic pressure of that cycle, and an increase in systolic pressure of the next. For patients in atrial fibrillation, several readings should be made and the arithmetic average of systolic and diastolic readings should be taken as, respectively, systolic and diastolic pressures.

4.5. Auscultatory gap

In some patients, especially in hypertension, the Korotkoff sounds disappear between the latter part of Phase I and Phase II, only to reappear at a lower pressure. Because of this phenomenon which is called the *auscultatory gap*, one can seriously underestimate the systolic, or overestimate the diastolic pressure. The error can be as high as 40 mmHg, and should be avoided by first estimating the systolic pressure by palpatory thods as described above.

4.6. Blood pressure reading in clinical shock

Due to low systemic pressure in shock, brachial artery pulsations and Korotkoff sounds may be greatly diminished or absent. This happens in the shock states caused by marked reduction in cardiac output (pump failure) or massive blood volume depletion (hemorrhage). Both of the above cause reflex contraction of blood vessels which increases peripheral vascular resistance thus reducing the blood flow especially in the extremities to such low levels that Korotkoff sounds can no longer be detected.

Under these circumstances, the indirect auscultatory blood pressure determination is so grossly inaccurate that it becomes meaningless. Direct blood pressure recording is the best method for monitoring these critically ill patients.

4.7. Indirect blood pressure reading in infants and children

The technique is similar to that used in adults, the only difference being in the size of the compression cuff. Muffling of Korotkoff sounds (Phase IV) and not the complete cessation of sound is the best index of diastolic pressure. As a general rule, the cuff should cover two-thirds of the arm above the elbow. Hence, small cuffs: 2·5, 5·8 and 12 cm wide should be available.

It is worth remembering that recent exercise may result in temporarily elevated blood pressure in all patients, including children. Crying may raise an infant's systolic pressure by as much as 30-50 mmHg.

Another problem is that the auscultatory sounds may be too faint to be heard in infants. In this situation, another indirect method for blood pressure determination, the so-called *flush method,* may be used. A suitable sphygmomanometer cuff is placed on the forearm or calf. The extremity is elevated and the limb distal to the cuff compressed by binding it firmly with an elastic bandage in order to empty it of blood. The cuff is then inflated to approx. 150 mmHg, the extremity lowered to the heart level and the bandage removed. The limb should appear very pale. The compression cuff pressure is then slowly released at a rate of 2-3 mmHg per second. The reading taken at the first appearance of a pink flush reflects the *mean,* not the systolic blood pressure.

4.8. Measurement errors

Instrument errors may be significant, especially in aneroid manometers. The use of inappropriate cuff sizes, too slow or too fast cuff deflation rate, and parallax of the dial, are other possible causes of error. Significiant errors may also be caused by sensory impairment, inattention or subconscious bias of the person measuring the blood pressure. The avoidance of errors in blood pressure reading is as important as the need for accurate diagnosis. Sphygmanometry leaves much to be desired, and biological variation in the same person further complicates the picture. This makes elimination of avoidable errors in measurement, all the more important.

4.9. Non invasive venous pressure estimation

The venous blood pressure reflects the *right atrial* (RA) *pressure,* and may be of important value in patients suffering right ventricular failure, right ventricular overload or constrictive or restrictive disorders affecting the right atrium and/or ventricle. Non-invasive assessment of venous pressure is particularly important when there are contra indications to invasive measurement or when there is difficulty using or inserting a venous catheter. Venous pressure is estimated by examination of the patient's neck veins.

Procedure:

- Lie the patient down, examine the neck and palpate the pulsation of the distende internal or external jugular veins.
- Sit the patient up.
- Note the disappearance of venous distention in the neck.
- Gradually lie the patient down again until filling of the vein can be observed.

- Using a centimeter ruler, measure the vertical distance between the middle of the right atrium and the neck level at the moment of filling up of the veins.

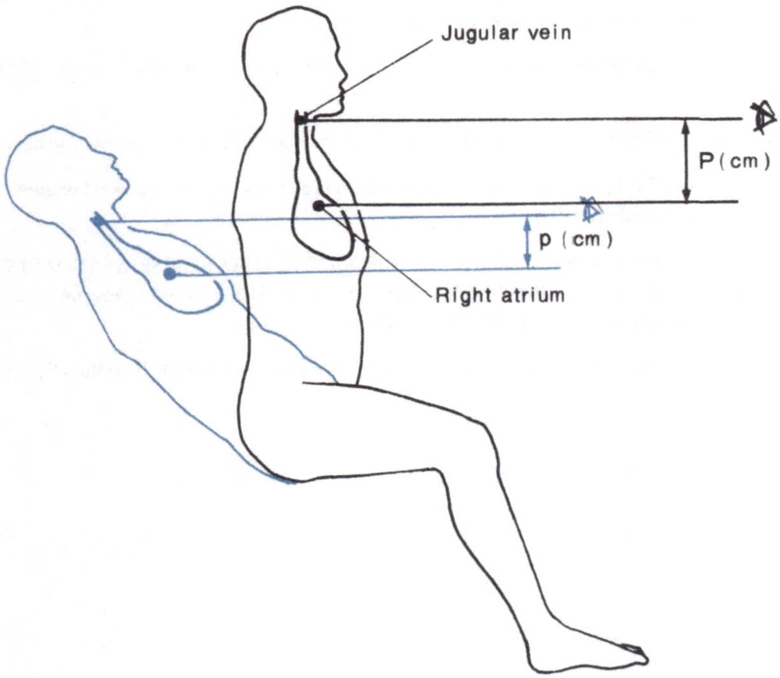

Fig. 8 - Non-invasive estimation of the venous pressure

4.10. Conclusions

This concludes our chapter on non-invasive blood pressure measurement. Less popular methods, including tonometry, automatic detection of Korotkoff sounds with automated cuff inflation and deflation, ultrasonic detection (Doppler) of arterial wall motion during cuff deflation, plethysmographic recognition of systolic blood pressure, etc., have not been discussed. The reader is referred to Bellville and Weaver's[6] chapter on blood pressure measurement for an account of the above methods.

The American Heart Association, in cooperation with an international panel of scientists, have published recommendations for human blood pressure determination by sphygmomanometry. In formulating these recommendations, direct blood pressure monitoring was used as the standart for the assessment of the factors governing the accuracy of sphygmomanometer method. It now is a well documented fact that while the direct method can be ± 1% or 1 mmHg accurate, the indirect auscultatory technique yelds a + 8 mmHg mean error in normal persons. The *validity* of the auscultatory technique is *so questionable* in patients in shock, that *direct pressure* monitoring is the *method of choice* in such cases.

BIBLIOGRAPHY

1. REPORT OF A SUBCOMMITTEE OF THE POSTGRADUATE EDUCATION COMMITTEE, AMERICAN HEART ASSOCIATION: "Recommendation for Human Blood Pressure Determination by Sphygmomanometers", *Circulation,* **36: 980-988**, 1967.

2. BAUM W.A. "Sphygmomanometers — Principles and Precepts", *Baum Co., publ., Copiague, N.Y.,* 1966.

3. BAUM W.A., "The Clinical Measurement of Blood Pressure", *Baum Co., publ., Copiague, N.Y.,* 1969.

4. BURCH, E.G., DE PASCALE, N.P.: "Primer of Clinical Measurement of Blood Pressure", *C.V. Mosby Co., publ., St Louis, Mo,* 1962.

5. COMMITTEE OF AMERICAIN HEART ASSOCIATION TO REVISE STANDARDISATION OF BLOOD PRESSURE READINGS: "Recommendation for Human Blood Pressure Determinations by Sphygmomanometers" *J.A.M.A.:* **147,7: 632-636**, 1951

6. BELLVILLE, J.W. AND WEAVER, CH. S.: "Techniques in Clinical Physiology", *MacMillan Co., London,* 1969.

V - DIRECT MEASUREMENT OF BLOOD PRESSURE

The word *direct* in the title of this chapter denotes a method of measurement based on direct contact of the measuring system with the bloodstream. The pressure measuring device (manometer and the like) is either introduced directly into a blood vessel or connected to it via fluid-filled tubes. The fluid in the tubes is incompressible and acts as a transmission medium for the blood pressure pulse. It is obvious that direct measurement of blood pressure is invasive; the skin and vessel wall are punctured to introduce part of the measuring system into the lumen of the blood vessel.

5.1. Choice of system

Two types of systems are used for direct pressure monitoring: *mechanical* and *electronic*. The mechanical systems, which are simple and relatively inexpensive are now giving way to more sophiscated electronic systems which have several advantages. They give hard copy recordings of pressure over a period of time, instantaneous systolic and diastolic values, and facilitate the remote monitoring of patients. The electronic systems also respond quickly and accurately to rapidly changing pressures.

After a short discussion of mechanical direct systems, the electronic monitoring of pressures and its medical applications will be reviewed.

5.1.1. Mechanical direct pressure system

A mercury or aneroid manometer is connected, via a fluid-filled catheter and air-filled space in a syringe (optional) to a lumen of a vessel.

The direct pressure values are obtained by visual readout of the height of a mercury column, or of a manometer dial. The large inertia (the reluctance to change velocity) of the volume of saline and mercury, and the compliance of the air-filled space, result in the inability of these systems to respond to fast changes in pressure. Hence, mechanical systems can only measure accurately so-called "average" or mean pressure.

Mechanical direct blood pressure monitoring is best suited for clinical situations in which the changes in pressure take place over several seconds, for example in venous blood, CSF or amniotic fluid pressure monitoring. In monitoring central venous pressure, it is advisable to use a mechanical system with the flushing arrangement, in order to prevent the formation of blood clots within intravascular cannulae. For cerebrospinal or amniotic fluid pressure monitoring, the flushing system *must not* be used. In CSF monitoring, there is no clotting problem and flushing may cause a dangerous pressure build up in the cerebral ventricular system.

5.1.2. Electronic direct pressure system

The most commonly used direct electronic pressure monitoring systems use three basic components:

- *Catheter:* a semi-rigid tube filled with fluid.
- *Transducer:* a device to convert mechanical force to an electric signal.
- *Monitor:* a device to amplify, condition, measure and display electric signals.

Plate 4 depicts the general arrangement of these components for direct monitoring.

The purpose of an effective direct pressure monitoring system is to reproduce visually, and measure the varying pressure waveform with minimal distortion. The system begins with the fluid-filled catheter or cannulae, which is introduced into the artery or vein. The catheter is connected to a semi-rigid plastic tube which transmits the pressure pulse from the catheter tip to the transducer.

For monitoring the arterial pressure, the catheter tip is usually inserted into one of the peripheral arteries, e.g., radial artery, by arterial puncture. For the measurement of venous and pulmonary artery pressures, the catheter tip is inserted into the radial, jugular or subclavian vein, which requires venous puncture.

5.2. Advantages of direct blood pressure measurement

Direct blood pressure measurement gives:

Good accuracy of pressure measurement.

Enhanced reliability in shock.

Availability of beat-to-beat measurements.

Availability of objective hard-copy time course recording.

Availability of true mean pressures.

Possibility of measurements at internally located sites.

Ease of telemetry.

Good fidelity recording during rapid changes of pressures.

With the increased reliability and sophistication of electronic instruments and the development of plastic catheters and heparin to prevent clotting, direct, continuous pressure monitoring has become part of the management of the seriously ill patient. It provides health personnel with better than ever assessment of patient condition and may lead to appropriate and sometimes life-saving therapy.

VI - OPERATION OF ELECTRONIC PRESSURE TRANSDUCERS AND CATHETERS

6.1. The transducer

Over the last 250 years, the direct methods of measuring blood pressure have been modified and improved. Cumbersome column manometers have been replaced by high fidelity, fast-response electro-mechanical transducer. The goose quills and trachea of Hale's day have been replaced by plastic tubing and, similarly, smoked drums and floating styluses have given way to electrical amplifiers, strip chart recorders and display screens. Nevertheless, the general principle has remained the same: direct puncture and cannulation of the blood vessel, and connection via a column of liquid to a pressure display device (manometer). To enable the electrical display and recording of pressure, a transducer is required to convert the mechanical pressure (i.e. force) into an electrical signal (voltage).

A key component of the transducer is the diaphragm. In its simplest form, it is a thin, flexible, circular plate. When the pressure is higher on one side, this plate deflects away from the higher pressure. In order to measure these deflections, (which, incidentally, are very small) a system of wires called a strain gauge is attached to the diaphragm. The principle of the strain gauge is that when a wire is stretched, its electrical resistance increases. On the contrary, if the wire is compressed, its resistance decreases. To render such changes in resistance more readily measurable, the wires are usually arranged in pairs to form a Wheatstone bridge. This means that as one pair of wires is being stretched by the diaphragm, a corresponding pair is compressed by the same movement. These changes of resistance are translated into changes of electric voltage, as the transducer bridge is powered by an external source (Fig. 9).

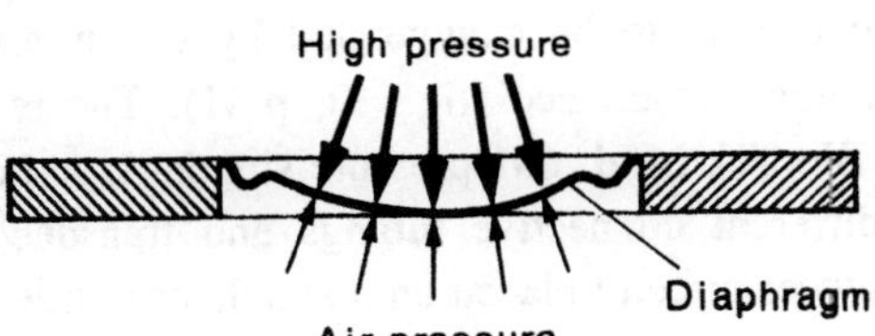

Fig. 9 - Principle of the pressure transducer

Typically, the output voltage of the transducer bridge is of the order of 50 microvolts per 1 mmHg of pressure difference across the transducer diaphragm. The transducer strain-gauge bridge is usually powered by an alternating voltage of 10 V.

Therefore, electrical signals are produced, which are proportional to the pressure difference across the diaphragm. As one side is vented to the atmosphere and the other exposed to the fluid (e.g. blood) at the site of pressure measurement, it constitutes a perfect arrangement for direct pressure measurement, with reference to the atmosphere, i.e. the conventional reference for medical pressure measurements.

6.2. Connecting tubing and catheters

External pressure transducers are the most commonly used, and to facilitate their connection to the point of measurement (e.g. artery, vein, body cavity, etc.) a plastic semi-rigid tubing is used. This is filled with fluid in order to transmit the pressure from the point of measurement to the transducer diaphragm. As we remember from Pascal's Law (see ch. 2), the pressure at the transducer end of the tubing will be the same as at the point of measurement, providing that the tubing is fully filled with fluid without any air spaces, that its walls are rigid and that both ends are positioned at the same level. If there is a difference in level between the ends of tubing, the hydrostatic pressure is added (or substracted). This may cause significant observer error if not accounted for and corrected.

6.3. Distortion of pressure

Air spaces or bubbles within the fluid-filled tubing act as a cushion for the pressure, because air is highly compressible. Pascal's Law (Ch. 2, p. 19), stating that pressure distribution in a non-compressible fluid is uniform, does not hold in this case and severe distortion of the pressure wave will occur.

A simular effect is observed when the walls of the connecting tubing are soft and extendable—hence the reason for semi-rigid walled tubing.

The volume displacement due to flexing of the diaphragm within the transducer also influences the distortion of pressure readout, and the length and diameter of the tubing also play a role.

What does all this mean? It means that the fluid-filled connecting system significantly influences what is observed as blood pressure. The slowly changing components of the pressure pulse are the ones likely to be reproduced most faithfully but the fast components tend to be exaggerated by the system. This is due to the phenomenon of mechanical resonance (fig. 10, p.41). The recordings in this figure were made using the Bio-Tek Mod. 601 pressure simulator and comparing the pressure pulse recorded via different connective tubings and transducers, with the pressure recorded from a transducer directly placed on a simulator (''true pressure''). From this, the following conclusions may be drawn: in order to reduce errors in measurements and monitoring of blood pressure pulses, use the shortest possible lengh of connective tubing between transducer and blood vessel (not more than 4' or 120 cm), elimitate all air bubbles from the system, and use small displacement transducers (less than 0·1 mm^3 per 100 mmHg of pressure).

Readers wishing to learn more about these problems of mechanical resonance and damping in the tubes and catheters used in blood pressure monitoring, are referred to the article by Latimer[1] and to chapter in Bruner's book[2].

6.4. Clotting problems and continuous flushing

Since blood pressure monitoring may be required for several days, the formation

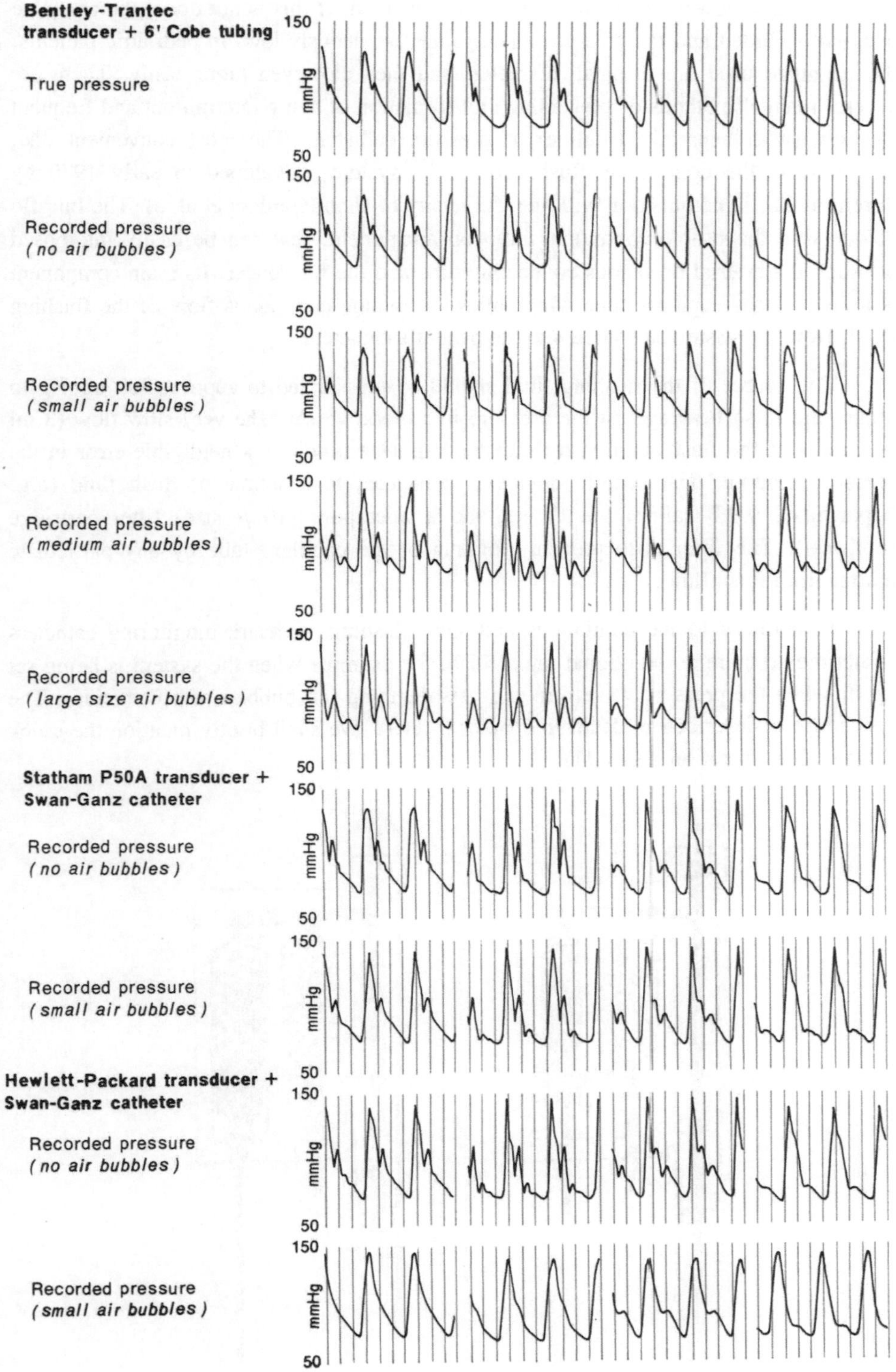

Fig. 10 - Arterial pressure waveforms distortions under different conditions

of blood clots indwelling cannulae must be prevented. If this is not done, the cannulae become occluded and the pressure readings are erroneously low. In pedriatric patients, the cannulae used are of small diameter, and they clot even more easily. There are several manual methods of preventing clot formation utilizing intermittent and frequent flushing (with heparinized saline) of pressure catheters. The most convenient one, however, is the continuous flush Intraflo ™ system, developed in early 1970 by Sorensen Co. in conjunction with the University of Utah (Gardner et al. [3]). The Intraflo device is a disposable continuous infusion attachment, that can be easily interposed between the arterial or venous connecting tube and the transducer. Its main component is a small glass capillary tube which allows a minute continuous flow of the flushing fluid, from a pressurized source into the patient's catheter.

The source of the flushing fluid should be pressurized to approx. 300 mmHg to assure the flush flow against the pressure in a blood vessel. The very slow flow (3 ml per hour) of the flush solution through the cannulae produces a negligible error in the pressure readout. The Intraflo device is connected to a source of flush fluid (e.g. heparinized 0·9% saline) via IV set and a micrapore (10 μ size) filter cartridge (optional). The filter is to prevent clogging of the capillary tube by any particulate matter from flush fluid.

In addition to the continuous and slow flushing, pressure monitoring catheters sometimes require an additional rapid flush, for example when the system is being set up or when the pressure waveform suggests damping (air bubbles or obstruction). The procedure is described in detail in chapter 8. Here, we shall briefly mention the quick flush valve operation (Fig. 11).

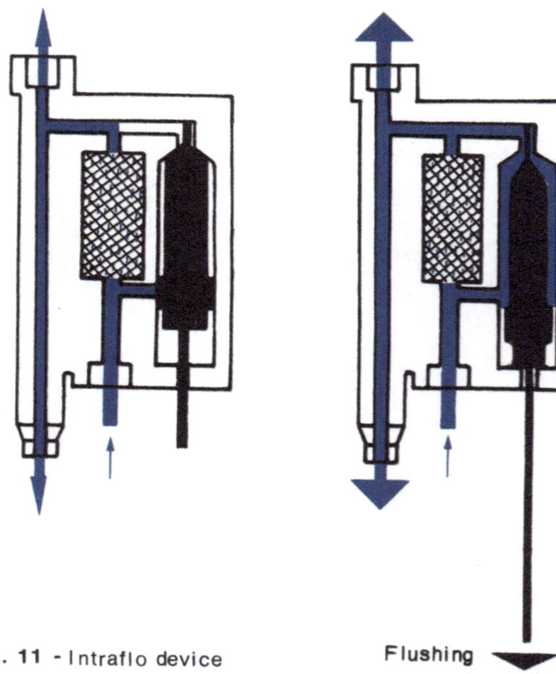

Fig. 11 - Intraflo device

The valve, which is normally closed, consists of a conical rubber plunger seated in the bypass channel shunting the capillary. The thin stem of the valve sticks outside the Intraflo and serves as a control. By pulling back on the valve stem, the plunger opens the bypass channel, temporarily opening the pressure monitoring line to the pressurized source of flush fluid. On releasing the stem, the rubber plunger immediately seals off the bypass path. The automatic closing of the valve, provides an extra safety measure against the whole volume of flushing fluid running rapidly into the patient's circulation.

When the automatic continuous flush system is used, extra care is necessary to eliminate all the air bubbles from the system, prior to starting the pressure monitoring procedure.

BIBLIOGRAPHY

1. LATIMER, K.E.: "The Transmission of Sound Waves in Liquid-Filled Catheter Tubes Used for Intravascular Blood Pressure Recording", *Med. & Biol. Eng.* **6:29-42**, 1968.

2. BRUNER, J.M.R.: "Handbook of Blood Pressure Monitoring", *PSG Publ. Co., Littleton, Ma.* 1978.

3. GARDNER, R.M. WARNER H.R., TORONTO A.F., GAISFORD, W.D.: "Catheter Flush System for Continuous Monitoring of Central Arterial Pulse Waveform", *Jo. Appl. Physiology* **29·6:911-913,** 1970.

VII - OPERATION OF ELECTRONIC MONITORS

The electrical voltage from the transducer varies according to changes (e.g. pulsatile) of the pressure in the blood vessel to which it is connected via a cannulae. Such voltage changes are very small, a few thousandths of a volt or less, and in order to visualize them an electronic monitor is needed. The monitor also provides energizing voltage for the transducer bridge. The monitor *amplifies* the small voltages from the transducer by a factor of at least 1000. The amplified voltage in turn deflects the electron beam in the cathode ray tube (CRT) causing changes in the position of the lighted trace on its screen. Such a *display* is continuous and provides information regarding the pressure levels as well as the pressure versus time graphic relationship known as the pressure waveform. In addition, the monitor may be equipped with *digital readouts,* pressure alarms, etc. This are the essentials of the electronic monitor but there are some points which are useful to know to avoid the pitfalls of Murphy's Law. (''If anything can go wrong, it will'': Arthur Bloch, Price, Stern & Sloan Publ., Los Angeles, 1977).

First of all, the monitor will work better if you plug it in, and secondly you can make it work if you fiddle with it long enough! The object of this chapter is to facilitate working with the monitor.

7.1. The pressure amplifier

As previously stated, very small voltages produced by the pressure transducer must he boosted (i.e. amplified) before they can be displayed on the monitor screen or readout. The pressure amplifier has an input jack to which the transducer is connected. At least two pins of this jack are the source of energizing voltage for the transducer, without which the strain gauge transducer cannot produce a signal, regardless wether or not changes in pressure occur across its diaphragm. Two or three other pins serve as voltage sensing imputs for the amplifier. If there is no voltage at these inputs the amplifier should produce no voltage at the output. It is regrettable that transducer cables of some manufacturers do not necessarily fit the connectors of the pressure amplifier of a different manufacturers as there is no standardization in the industry. As a rule it is wise to remember that the transducers and transducer cables must be compatible with the brand and type of monitor pressure amplifier.

7.2. Front panel controls

Here is the list of most common controls:

1 - zero

2 - gain or sensitivity

3 - pressure range (scale)

4 - calibration

5 - test

6 - instantaneous/mean pressure readout

7 - alarm level(s)

8 - alarm OFF/active/reset/status indicators.

There is an increasing tendency to reduce the total number of controls for operational simplicity. The feat is accomplished by substituting previous manual controls with automatic ones. They have not, however, disappeared completely in a functional sense, so an explanation is in order.

7.3. "Zero"

The "zero" control ensures that the amplifier output readout shows zero when there is zero pressure at the transducer. This means that both sides of the transducer should be at atmospheric pressure. Even a small unbalancing in the strain gauge system within the transducer, or a minute permanent deformation of its diaphragm will result in a non-zero signal with zero pressure difference. This can, and should be electrically compensated for by using the zero control knob while venting the transducer dome (see vent stopcock position in chapter 8) to the atmosphere, separated from other sources of non-zero pressure (e.g. patient line flush system). Some amplifiers have this zero control in the form of a rotating knob, others as a push-switch to activate automatic zeroing routine within the amplifier. The principle is the same in both: the transducer open to air *must* produce *zero* readout on the display (i.e., trace at zero level and zero ± 1 mmHg on the digital readout). On some monitors the automatic zeroing procedure takes up to 10 seconds, i.e., only after this time do the displays in use read zero.

7.4. Gain

The *gain* (sensitivity) control on the pressure amplifier is to adjust the magnitude of beam or pen deflection during the pressure measurements. The minute voltages appearing on the output of the transducer are in accord with the pulsations of its diaphragm. It is important that each change in pressure across the diaphragm produce corresponding change in the voltage. Such changes must be linear and consistent. A linear relationship allows accurate and fairly easy electronic measurement of the pressure because each incremental change in pressure always produces the same incremental change in voltage (within the pressure measuring range). Consistency of measurements is also important.

The hospital ward or intensive care unit is a fast-paced, high-tension environment, to which present-day transducers are poorly suited. A delicate diaphragm is essential for adequate sensitivity. The inadvertent distortion of this fragile element due to mechanical shock or over-pressure cause the need of frequent amplifier calibration, zero and gain adjustment. In addition, both the strain gauge and amplifier elements are not perfectly thermally stabilised and their parameters change with time due to variations in ambient temperature. It is good practice to allow ample warmup time (ca. 30 minutes) before measurements are made.

Nevertheless, both the zero and gain functions should be checked frequently (preferably every 4-8 hours) to assure the accuracy of the system. A detailed description of checking procedures is in the next chapter.

Some recent pressure monitoring amplifiers may have this control of gain/sensitivity completely removed from the front panel. For the sake of operational simplicity such amplifiers are limited to use of precalibrated or standardized transducers. Many presently marketed pressure transducers have a voltage-to-pressure conversion factor equal to 50 microvolts/mmHg+10Venergizing voltage. The pressure amplifiers with preset gain will only operate properly when connected to these standardized transducers. They remain standardized as long as they are not physically damaged. They (as well as non-standardized transducers) should therefore be handled with extreme care. Dropping one on a hard floor will almost certainly almost certainly result in complete damage or in the loss of sensitivity and zero calibration.

The calibration switch works with the gain/sensitivity control. When depressed, it delivers a voltage at the amplifier input which corresponds to a predermined pressure value (e.g. 100 mmHg). This value is a "magic" cal-factor supplied by the manufacturer for a given transducer-amplifier combination. The cal-factor number should be displayed when the cal-button is depressed and when there is *no* pressure signal on the transducer (open to air). If the displayed value is different two things can be wrong: the transducer has "lost" its sensitivity matching or the amplifier has the wrong gain adjustment. In the second case, the remedy is simple: readjust the gain control on the amplifier. However, there is no way of knowing this fact in advance, especially as the first possibility may be (and most likely is) the problem. The best way to assess the situation and find the true cal-factor of the transducer is to perform the physical test against a mercury column manometer as described in chapter 8.

7.5. Range set

The pressure range control (scale) is usually in the form of a lever switch with two or more positions (e.g., 30, 60, 300 mmHg). At the highest range setting, for example 300 mmHg, a pressure of this value when "seen" by the transducer will produce a fullscale trace deflection on the face of the CRT in the monitor. The same applies for the respective lower range scales. This scale change switch enables observation of pressure waveforms in the lower as well as higher pressure levels. For example: the 300 mmHg range is well suited for measurement of arterial pressure, but for central venous or pulmonary artery pressure a range of 30 mmHg is much more appropriate. This range switch can be deleted and substituted by a push-button stepwise control or automatic programmable range in the most modern equipment. In either case, the actual pressure range is displayed on the CRT or elsewhere.

7.6. Function switch

The instantaneous/mean pressure readout control is a switch or switches controlling both the digital readout of pressure value and the CRT display. They are frequently used for switching the readouts to display either systolic, diastolic or mean pressure and sometimes S/D (systolic-diastolic) alternately. In the instantaneous function, the amplifier samples the values of maximum systolic and minimum diastolic pressures and displays them in numerical form in a readout window or screen. In the mean position, the amplifier perfoms a mathematical integration resulting in averaging of the pressure pulse. The mean value will then be displayed graphically on the screen and as a numerical readout. It is probable that all of these values will be displayed on the CRT screen when the new generation of monitors reaches the market so obviating the need for a separate control for switching instantaneous to mean pressures.

7.7. Alarms

The alarm controls represent an additional feature in some models of pressure amplifier. The alarm is usually a beeper signal combined with a light indicator. The amplifier activates the alarm if and when the pressure exceeds either the high or low limit values for more than 5 seconds. The high and low limits can be preset manually by the control knobs or slides. In future generations the presetting of alarm levels will be accomplished electronically. The alarm sounds until the unit deliberately reset by the operator. This usually also involves medical intervention or change in alarm levels.

7.8. Summary of an ideal amplifier

In summary, the object of the pressure amplifier is to provide a calibrated and linear over the entire pressure-proportional signal measurement range. The zero and gain drifts in the amplifier should be negligible. The accuracy of the pressure measurement system should be ± 1 mmHg and the rapidity of response to changes in voltage (pressure) should be a least 0·6 v/m sec. The essential controls on the amplifier are:
— zero (preferably push-in),
— test (push-in),
— alarm activate/reset.

The other controls are hand-downs from previous technology and will be gradually replaced by automatic devices.

7.9. The pressure writer (recorder)

Direct writing devices is the traditional method of display. Contemporary writers operate on the same principle as the previously (chapter 1) described smoked drum kymograph. 20th century electronics, mechanics and chemistry contributed convenient features. The direct writers reproduce the pressure waveform on a strip of paper using electromechanical, fast reponse, pens. The parper speed is usually 25 mm/sec (sometimes 12·5, 50 or 100 mm/sec). This speed must be constant. Thus rectilinear movement of the voltage-driven pen produces the pressure display vs. time on the paper. Direct writers usually require some controls, notably trace position and paper speed selector. Again, as with the amplifiers, modern engineering designs tend to reduce the number and operational complexity of controls to the bare minimum. The newest generation of direct writers has automatic trace positioning but paper speed selection is either deleted or left to the operator.

7.10. The CRT display

The CRT letters signify Cathode-Ray-Tube. The CRT display uses luminescent phosphor on its face screen to visualize a trace. The phosphor lights when it is hit by an electron beam. The moving strip of paper of the direct writer is replaced here by a moving electron beam across the screen. Conventionally the beam moves horizontally at a steady speed from left to right (so-called time-base). The horizontal speed of the time-base beam is 12·5 mm/sec or, more commonly, 25 mm/sec—i.e., the same as the speed of paper in direct writers. When the beam reaches the right edge of the screen it rapidly jumps back to the left side and resumes its sweep at the same steady pace. The voltages applied to the so-called vertical input of the CRT display produce vertical deflections of the continuously, horizontally travelling beam, thus "drawing" a curved line corresponding to the voltage changes as a function of time. As we described before, the pressure (a mechanical variable) is converted by the transducer into voltage (an electrical variable) and this voltage is magnified by means of an amplifier. Thus the *vertical* deflections of the beam on the CRT screen are proportional to the instantaneous pressure values at the site of the catheter tip.

There are two basic varieties of CRT display: "bouncing ball" and "solid trace". While the former is less expensive in terms of initial outlay it only provides a continuous display of approx. 1 second of moving "window" on the pressure waveform. This is due to limited persistency of the luminous phosphor on the screen. When the spot on the phosphor is hit by the electron beam, a luminous dot is produced which gradually fades away after 1 second, unless it is hit by the beam again (refreshed). The latter, "Solid trace" display, does just that, i.e. refreshes rapidly all points hit by the beam during its basic sweep across the screen. A memory function is required to identify the points to be refreshed. Recent advances en computer technology have provided a solution to this problem in the form of a shift register and at a reasonable cost. While the "solid trace" display is more expensive (additional components) it provides a much more convenient and precise readout. In effect it produces a trace of constant luminosity across the entire screen. Depending then on the screen *size* and the speed of time-base, the pressure wave may be displayed in a time window of 4 to 8 seconds as a solid luminous trace moving across the screen. The time convention is preserved, as in a bouncing ball display, i.e., the earliest events are to the left on the screen, the most recent, to the right.

In a sense the solid trace display produces a result similar to the direct writer except that it continuously disappears to be replaced by the most recent waveform. This is done of course *without* producing the reams of paper as would be the case in continuous pressure monitoring using a direct writer. Futhermore, the solid trace can be "frozen" on the screen at the operator's command or alarm activation in order to preserve the fragments and events of particular interest for study, diagnosis and a permanent record. This is accomplished by writing out the "frozen" waveform from the screen on the direct writer when available. In effect then, by combining the solid trace display with freeze and alarm options the ultimate convenience in pressure monitoring can be achieved: continuous pressure readout on the screen combined with hard-copy record of events of interest.

The CRT solid-trace display is the strate-of-the-art device enabling a continuous readout of multiple pressure channels combined on a single screen. This is all accomplished at reasonable cost and great convenience when compared with the continuous direct writers.

Visual inspection of the pressure pulse contour as it is displayed on the CRT not only provides direct information on the patient but also affords continuous assessment of the *quality* of the measurement itself. As mentioned in chapter 6, the pressure reading becomes severely distorted if, for example, there is an air bubble within the catheter, pressure tubing or transducer dome. This and other errors (see ch. 9) are easily identified by looking at the patterns displayed on the CRT. This fact is very important for the valid assessment of the pressure monitoring process and its usefulness to guide clinical interventions. Good and accurate CRT display is then *the most essential* component for pressure monitoring.

7.11. Display of pressure values

The values of pressure can be directly read off the CRT screen. While this is the preferred method, somewhat cumbersome calibration grids have to be placed (overlayed) on the screen itself. For convenience, most manufacturers do provide some sort of meter display to measure either *peak systolic* or *minimum diastolic* pressures. The readout may be either on a dial or by flashing lighted numbers. In both cases the peak pressure values are given directly in mmHg. These readouts are accomplished by automatic electronic measurement (peak-sample-and-hold technique) of the pressure pulse wave. The presently used electronic circuits do not have the ability to distinguish between a good quality and a poor trace and produce the numerical readout regardless. Hence such readouts must be used with great care, and only after controlling the *quality* of the tracing on the CRT. The indiscriminate use of digital displays alone without validation by CRT trace may lead to grave mistakes and consequences in clinical interventions.

The display of mean *pressure* is a valuable tool. It provides either dial or digital readout of the true electronic *average* of a pressure waveform. As we have mentioned (ch. 3), the derivation of mean value for the pressure pulse is a complex operation. The automatic electronic averaging is the most accurate and convenient way of obtaining the mean pressure. The continuous display of mean pressure yields valuable clinical information. A quality monitor will usually include the mean pressure display feature with either dial or digital display or a strip paper recorder, or both.

HUMAN BLOOD CIRCULATION: (SIMPLIFIED DIAGRAM)

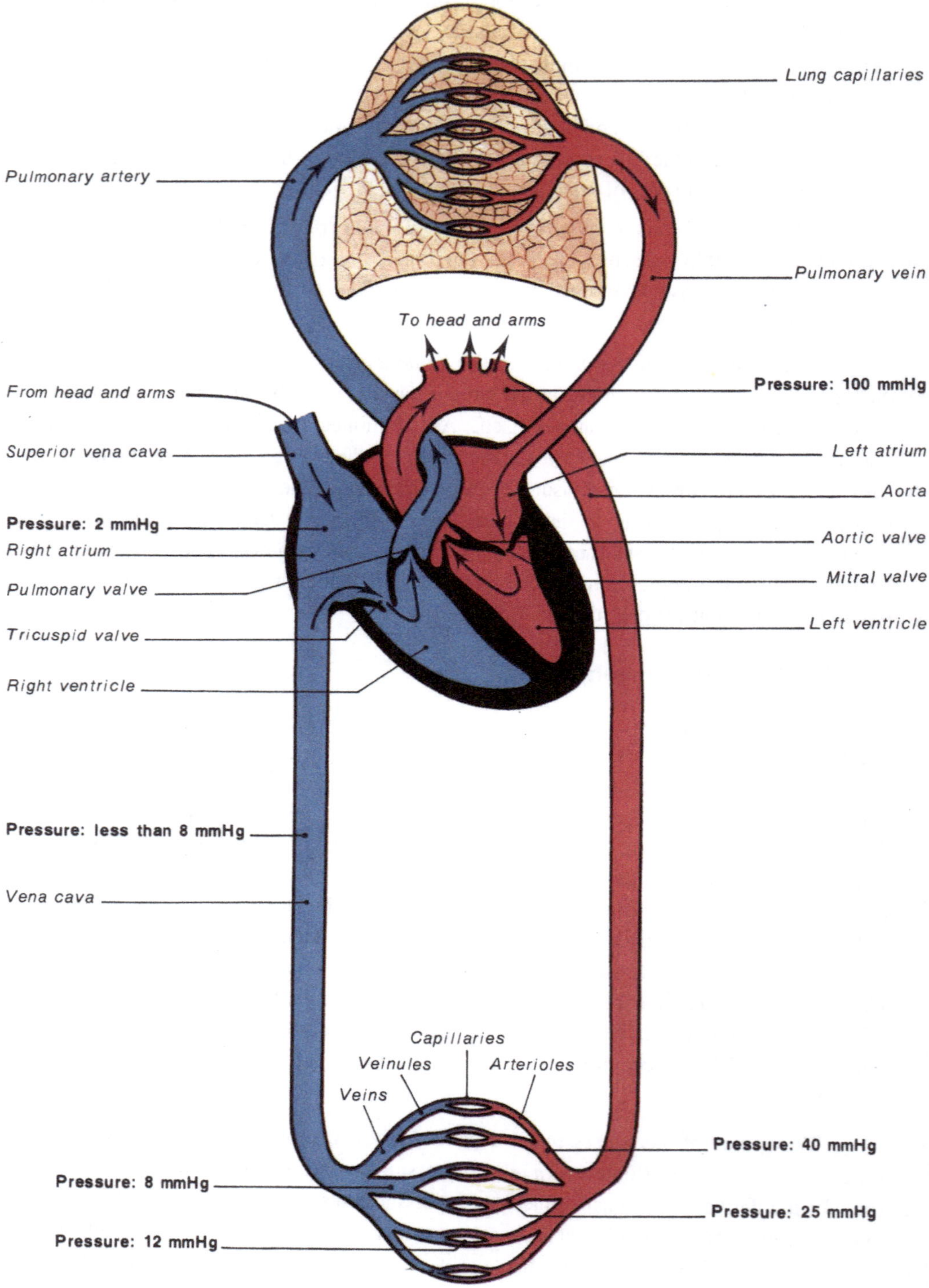

VIII - HOW TO PREPARE THE SYSTEM FOR DIRECT PRESSURE MONITORING

This chapter will deal with practical aspects of assembling, flushing and calibrating of the catheter-tubing-transducer-monitor-system.

8.1. Components for system with continuous flush

The components necessary to prepare one of the many monitoring system configurations, including the continuous flush feature, are illustrated on Plate 2.

Plate 3 shows the electronic monitor with all controls, CRT display, amplifier, alarms and readouts. Plate 4 illustrates the basic assembly of the system including items from Plates 2 & 3, plus IV pole and transducer holder.

Other auxiliary materials not shown on the plates:

- sterile male Luer-Lok caps;
- bottle of sterile water;
- 2 cc syringe;
- alcohol wipe pads;
- medication label.

8.2. How to assemble the system

To assemble the system as shown on Plate 4, the following step-by-step procedure is recommended: (''A'' in step numbers denotes Assembly).

Step A1. — Add 1000 units of Heparin to 500 ml infusion pack of 0·9 % sodium chloride. Knead the pack gently to mix.

Step A2. — Label infusion pack with date, time, contents and initials.

Step A3. — Invert infusion pack with outlets facing vertically upward.

Step A4. — Attach the pediatric IV set with roller clamp open to the infusion pack. Maintain sterility during attachment.

Step A5. — While holding the pack vertically, squeeze all air out from it. This is to prevent air from entering the catheter system once the heparinized solution is emptied from the infusion pack.

Step A6. — Suspend the infusion pack on the IV pole.

Step A7. — Fill drip chamber of pediatric IV set 1/4 full and close the roller clamp temporarily.

Step A8. — Place pressure bag (with manometer) over the infusion pack.

Step A9. — Attach the other end of the IV set to flush connector of Intraflo (Pl. 4). Maintain sterility.

Step A10. — Connect the 3-way stopcock to the Intraflo outlet (Pl. 4) and cover its side port with a cap. Maintain sterility.

Step A11. — Connect the 36 ''or 48'' long pressure tubing to the Intraflo inlet.

Step A12. — Attach the translucent dome to a transducer. Maintain sterility.

Step A13. — Attach 3-way stopcock to a vertical outlet on the transducer dome. Maintain sterility.

Step A14. — Connect the transducer cable to the monitor.

Step A15. — Plug the monitor into a line outlet (if not already done). Switch power ON.

It is good practice to complete the above assembly procedure, especially the monitor connection and warmup for at least 30 minutes prior to the arrival of the patient. This will afford better stability of the monitor-transducer system while allowing for adequate warmup time.

Once the system is assembled, it is ready for priming, (i.e. filling) with fluid and flushing. As mentioned before it is necessary to fill all the tubes and connections between transducer diaphragm and the patient catheter attachment in order to be able to transmit the pressure from the vessel in a body to the transducer. This filling *must* be thorough and complete to avoid air spaces and bubbles within the system in order to prevent pressure wave distortions. Hence the need for thorough flushing of the system.

8.3. Filling and flushing the tubing/transducer system

A useful step-by-step procedure for flushing: (''F'' in the step numbers denotes Flush) is explained on Plates 5 through 10.

The last step (Plate 10 step F15) completes the priming and flushing procedure for direct arterial blood pressure monitoring system using continuous flush device. It is now the time (if not already done) to prepare the electronic monitor for action. After switching the power ON, the luminous traces should apprear on the CRT screen (Plate 11 Figure 1). The alarm switches on the monitor should be turned OFF (Plate 11 Figure 2). The high range and systolic pressure display functions (if applicable) (Plate 11 Figure 3) should be selected.

8.4. ''Level'', ''zero'', and ''calibrate'' the transducer

These procedures should be performed directly prior to insertion of the catheter into the patient's vascular (or other) system. The transducer position (level) with respect to the patient is essential, and this is usually adjusted while the patient is being prepared.

COMPONENTS FOR PRESSURE MONITORING SYSTEM WITH CONTINUOUS FLUSH

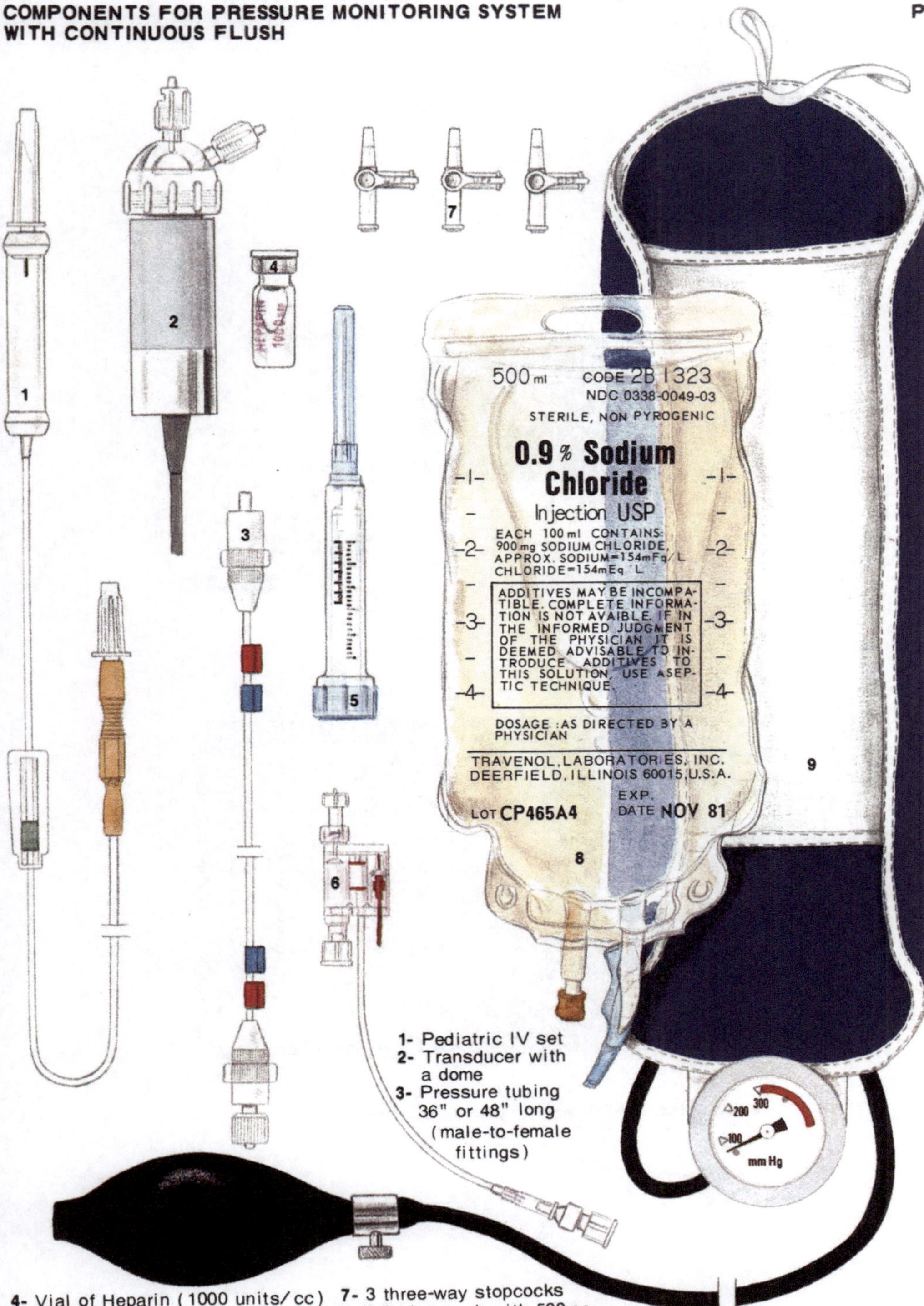

1- Pediatric IV set
2- Transducer with a dome
3- Pressure tubing 36" or 48" long (male-to-female fittings)
4- Vial of Heparin (1000 units/cc)
5- 3 cc syringe
6- Continuous flush device (Intraflo-Sorenson)
7- 3 three-way stopcocks
8- Infusion pack with 500 cc of 0.9% sodium chloride
9- Pressure bag with manometer and bulb pump

Monitor described in the text

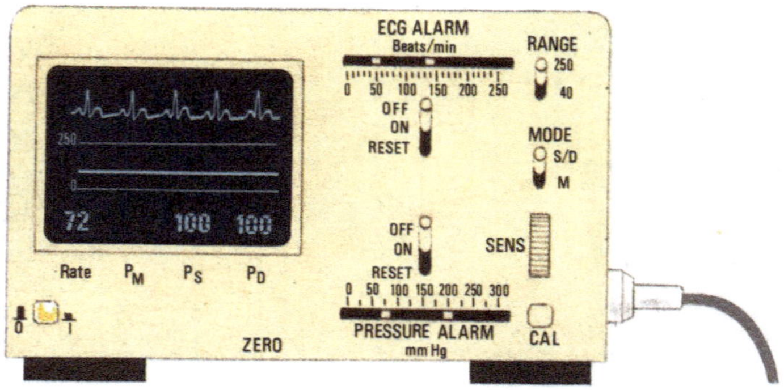

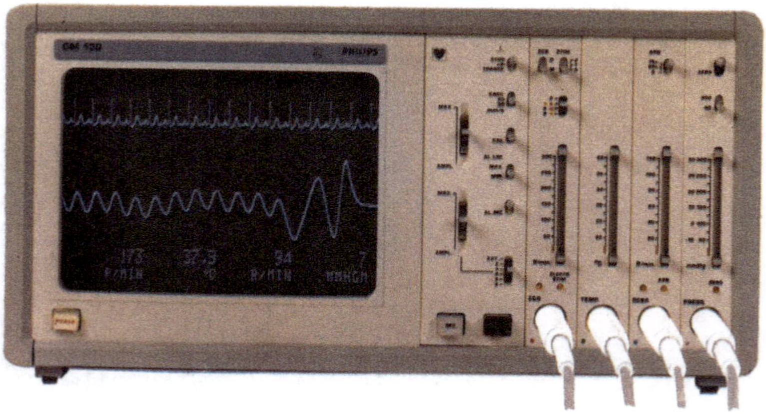

Philips Mod. CM 130 monitor with zero automatic

COMPLETE PRESSURE MONITORING SYSTEM

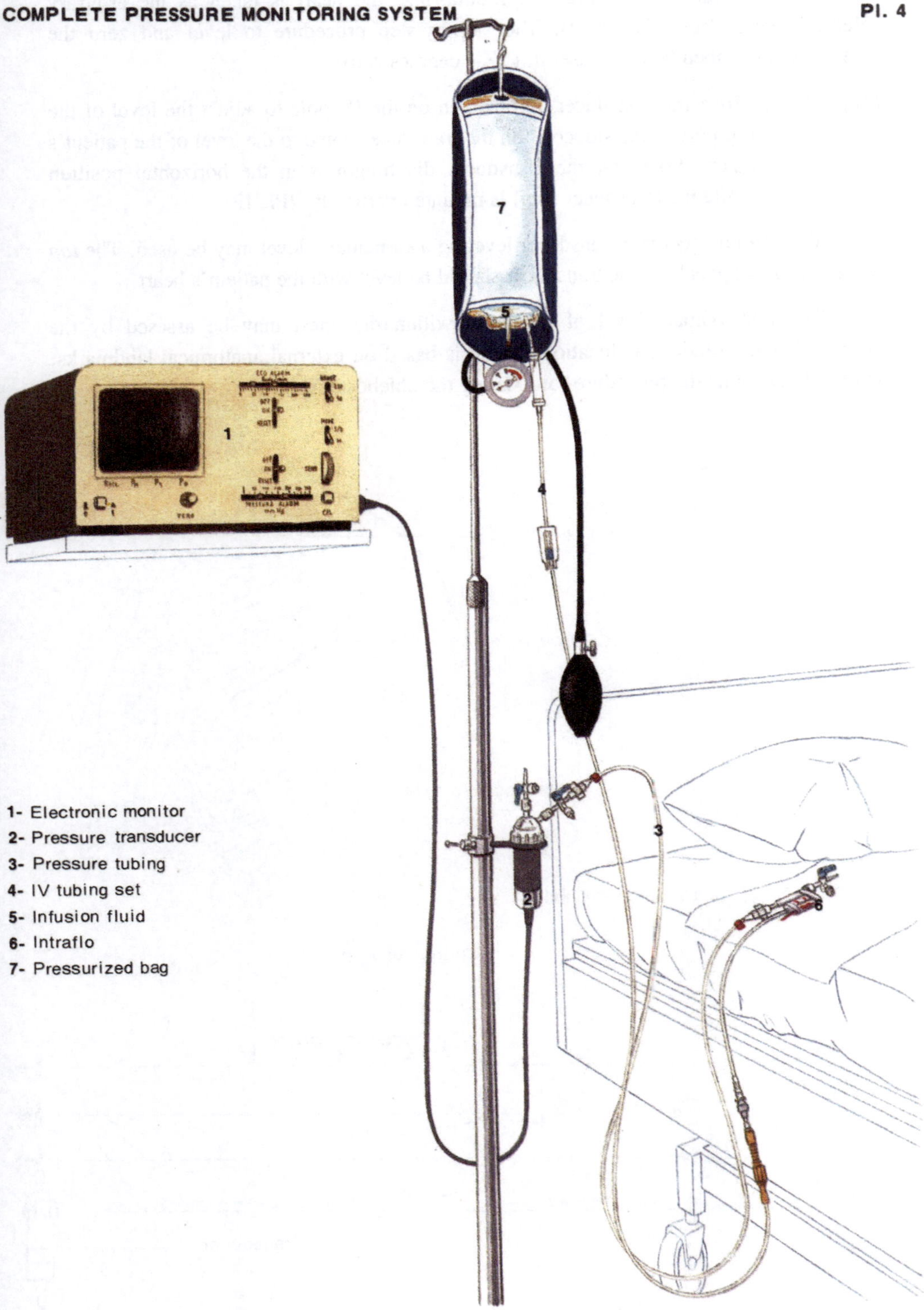

1- Electronic monitor
2- Pressure transducer
3- Pressure tubing
4- IV tubing set
5- Infusion fluid
6- Intraflo
7- Pressurized bag

In cardiovascular pressure monitoring, the heart is taken as the arbitrary reference level (see Chapter 2). The step-by-step procedure to level and zero the transducer described below is useful. (''Z'' denotes zero):

Step Z1. — Move the transducer up or down on the IV pole to adjust the level of the top port of the stopcock on the transducer dome to the level of the patient's heart. Note that the transducer diaphragm is in the horizontal position while the transducer itsefl is mounted vertically. (Pl. 12).

To facilitate accurate transducer leveling a carpenter's level may be used. The *top outlet* of the stopcock on the transducer should be level with the patient's heart.

The approximate level of the heart within the chest may be assesed by the so-called phlebostatic axis location, which is based on external anatomical landmarks. (Fig. 12) explains the procedure for locating the phlebostatic axis.

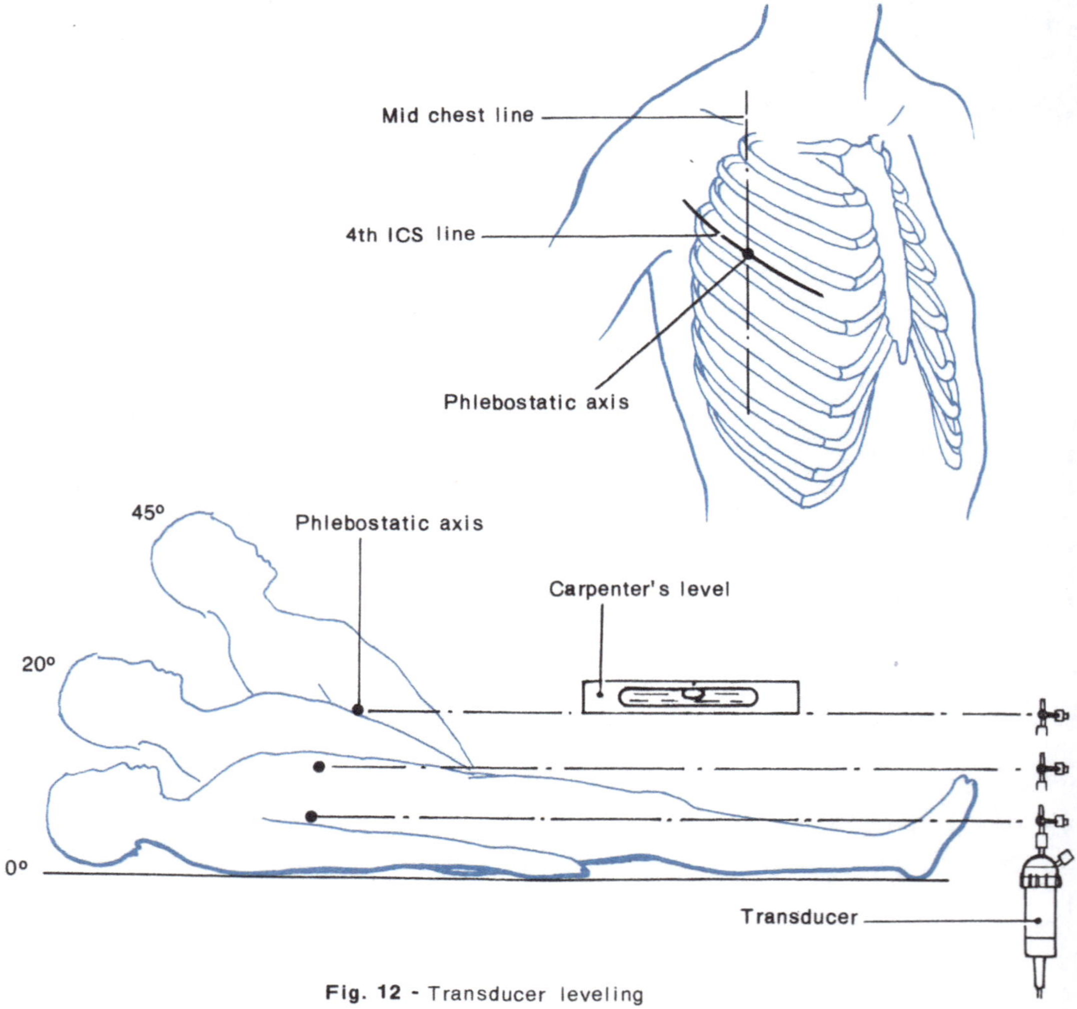

Fig. 12 - Transducer leveling

- Locate 4th sternal intercostal space (4th ICS).
- Trace imaginary circumferential line laterally at the level of the 4th ICS.
- Trace imaginary division line between anterior and posterior chest (mid chest line).
- The intersection of these two lines is the phlebostatic axis.

The purpose of leveling the transducer stopcock outlet port with the heart is to avoid the effects of hydrostatic pressure. Hydrostatic pressure causes erroneous pressure readings when the transducer is positioned above or below the heart level.

Blood pressure monitoring, as a rule, is performed simultaneously with ECG monitoring, hence the reason for multiple-trace display on CRT screen. If not already done, connect now the patient electrocardiogram monitoring electrodes to the monitor.

For step-by-step procedure in performing ''zero'' and ''calibration'' manœuvres follow the instructions on plates 13, 14 and 15.

8.5. Verification test

Although the entire system is now ready to start monitoring blood pressure, it is advantageous to double check that everything is working well. This may be accomplished by connecting the system to a source of a *known* pressure. The so-called physical verification test procedure does just that. This test may be performed not only prior starting monitoring (recommended) but also during the course of monitoring or whenever there is any doubt about the system performance or the clinical implication of pressure values obtained during monitoring. Transducers are very delicate and often go out of calibration as a result of mechanical impact or even inadvertant overpressure in the system caused for example by blood sample withdrawal or a medication injection. Thus the physical test is a most important part of routine pressure monitoring practice.

Parts of a mercury column sphygmomanometer may be used as source of known pressure. The connections and the step-by-step procedure are shown on plates 16, 17, 18 and 19. Then follows. The letter ''T'' in step numbers denotes ''Test''.

Step T8. – (Optional). To make sure no air bubbles were introduced into the system a quick flush as described in steps F5-F11 (Plates 5, 6, 7, 8 and 9) is recommended.

If a mercury manometer is not readily obtainable, a physical test may be performed using the *height* of a water column (heparinized saline fluid can be used as it has virtually the same specific weight as water). For this purpose, an additional 36'' (approx. 1 m.) plastic IV tubing and a *metric* ruler (1 meter) are necessary. The flush infusion pack serves as the source of saline. The step-by-step procedure is illustrated on Fig. 8 plate 19.

This concludes the descriptions of all technical procedures for the preparation and testing of the system for continuous monitoring of arterial blood pressure. The variants of this system and procedures intended for monitoring the pressure of other body fluids (e.g. cerebrospinal and amniotic) will be described in Chapters 14, 15.

FLUSHING PROCEDURE

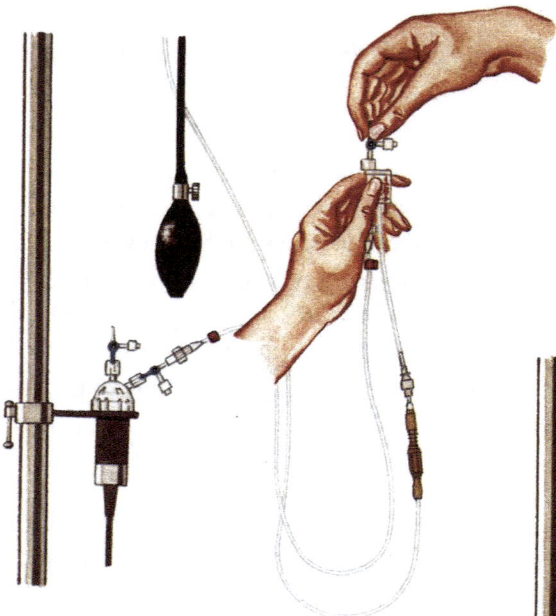

Step F 1. Turn the Intraflo stopcock, OFF to connection for patient.

Step F 2. Open the transducer to the pressure tubing by turning the stopcock on the side of the transducer dome.

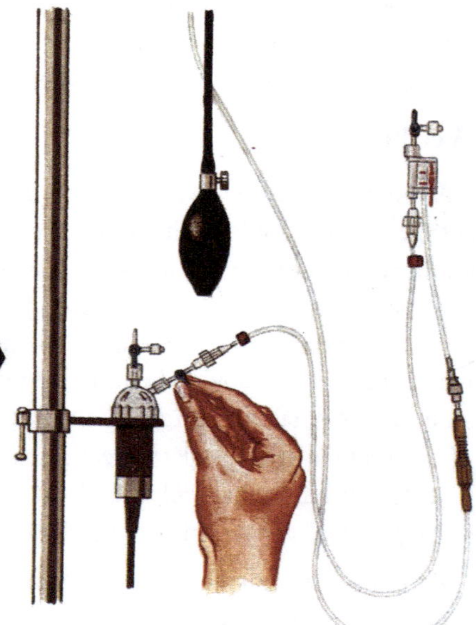

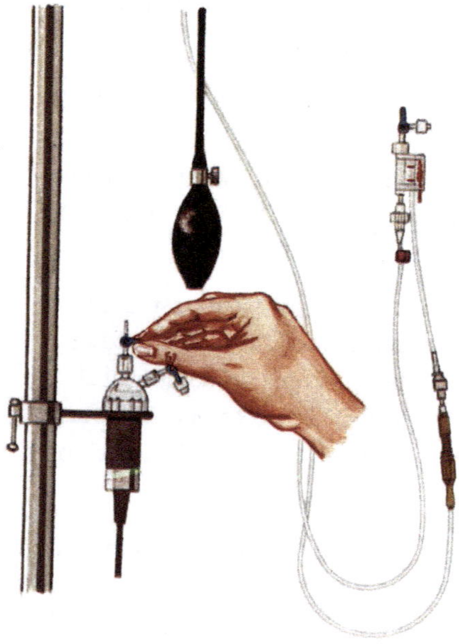

Step F 3. Open to air the vertical stopcock on the transducer dome.

Step F 4.

Pump air into pressure bag in order to pressurize infusion pack. The manometer should read 300 mmHg for arterial pressure monitoring or 150 mmHg for pulmonary artery pressure monitoring.

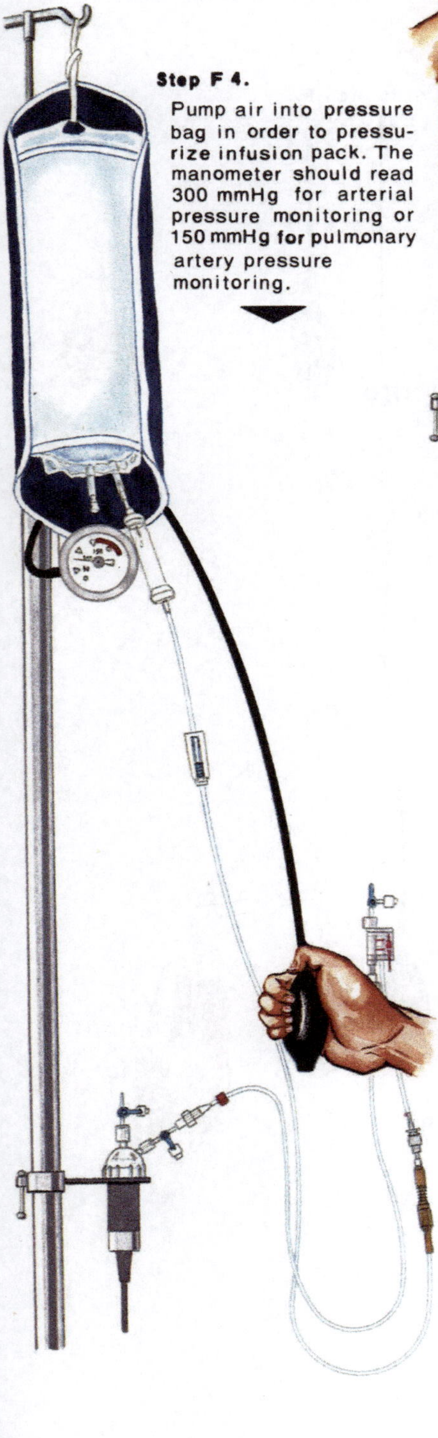

Step F 5.

Open roller clamp valve on the pediatric IV tubing.

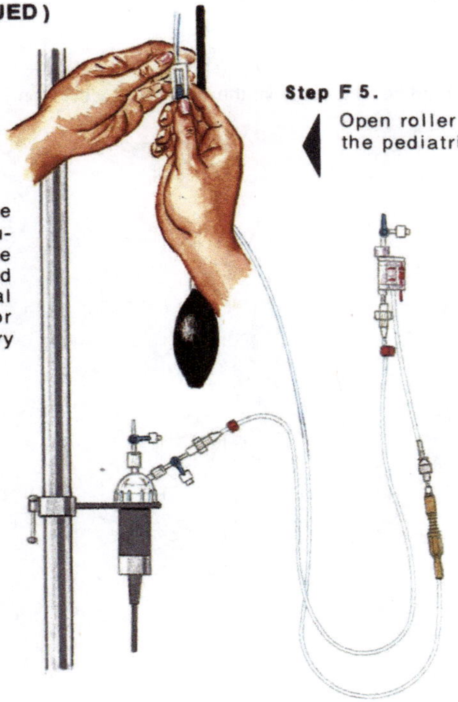

Step F 6. Pull out and **hold** the flush valve on Intraflo. The entire system should be filling with the fluid.

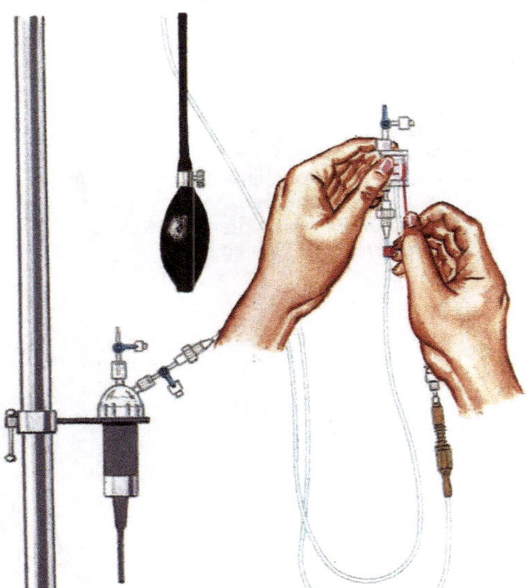

Step F 7 Is the fluid coming out from the vertical stopcock on the top of the transducer dome?

Continue

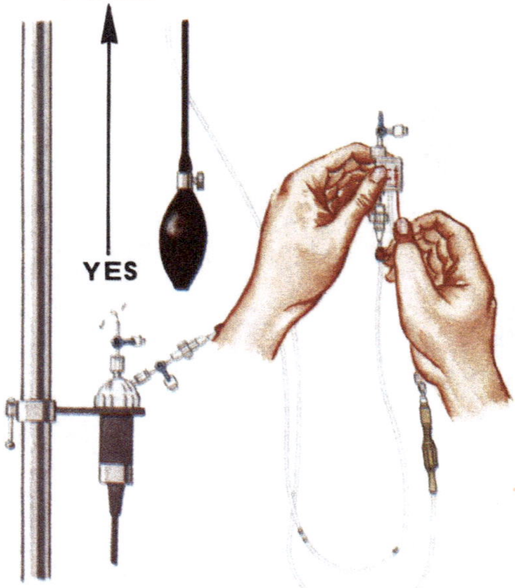

Return to step F 1

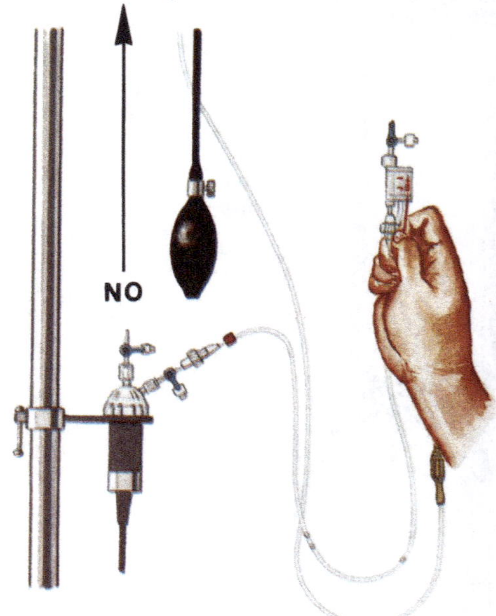

Step F 8.

Allow the fluid to flow out until **all air** bubbles are removed from the tubing. Tap gently on the elements of the system to facilitate removal of air bubbles. Bubbles will interfere with fidelity of pressure tracing.

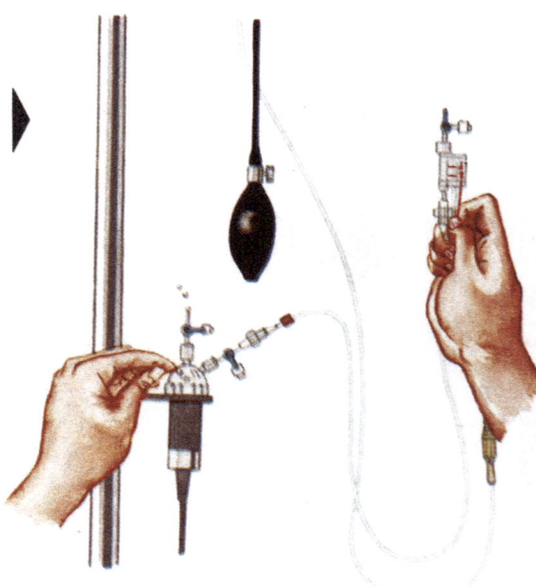

Step F 9.

Release the Intraflo flush valve to stop flow of the fluid.

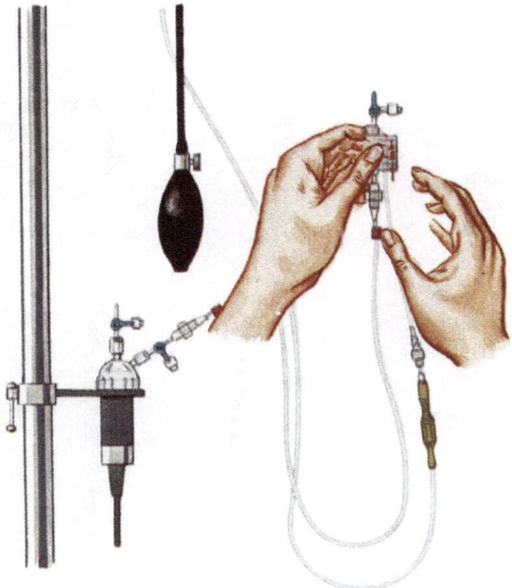

Repeat steps F 6-F 9

Step F 10.

Inspect the system.
Are there any bubbles?

YES

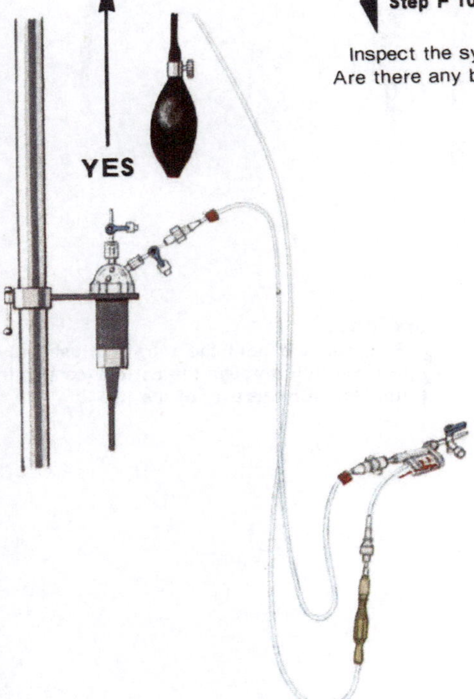

NO

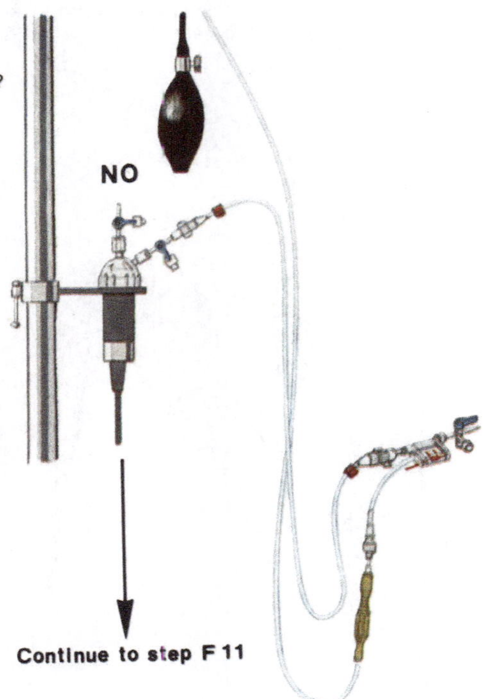

Continue to step F 11

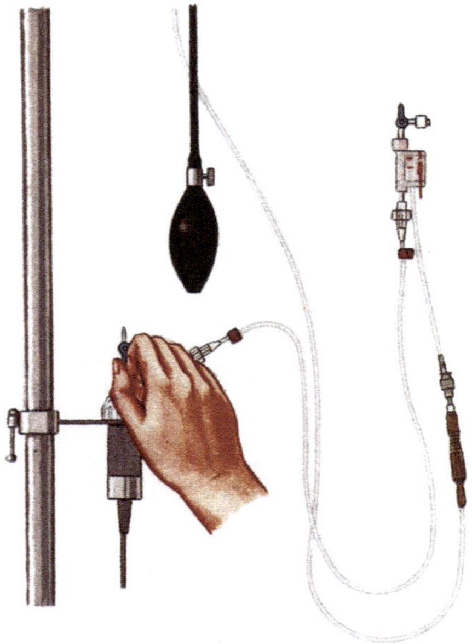

Step F 11. Turn OFF to air vertical stopcock on the transducer dome.

Step F 12. Turn the Intraflo stopcock to open the pressure tubing via Intraflo to the patient connect tip.

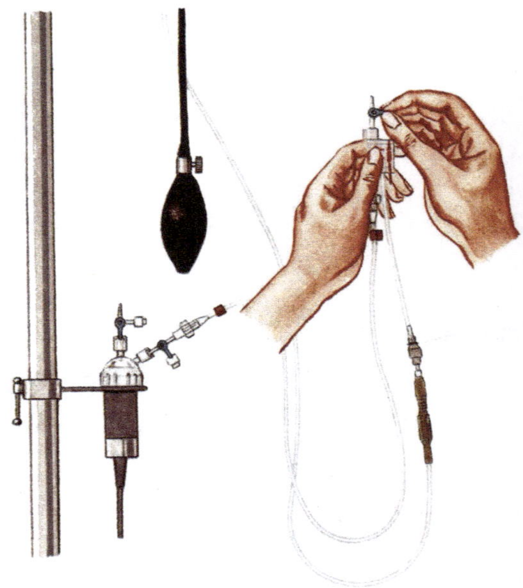

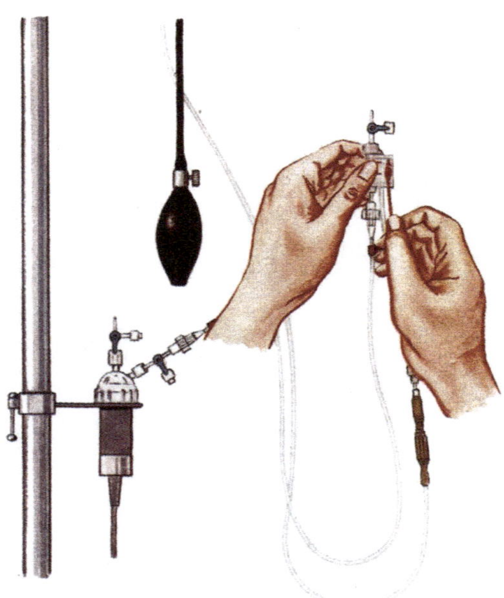

Step F 13.
Pull out and hold the Intraflo flush valve to force fluid through the patient connecting tip. Maintain sterility of the tip.

Step F 14. Verify that fluid is coming out from patient connection and there are no air bubbles in the short pressure tubing extension (if such is used between the Intraflo outlet and patient connecting tip).

YES

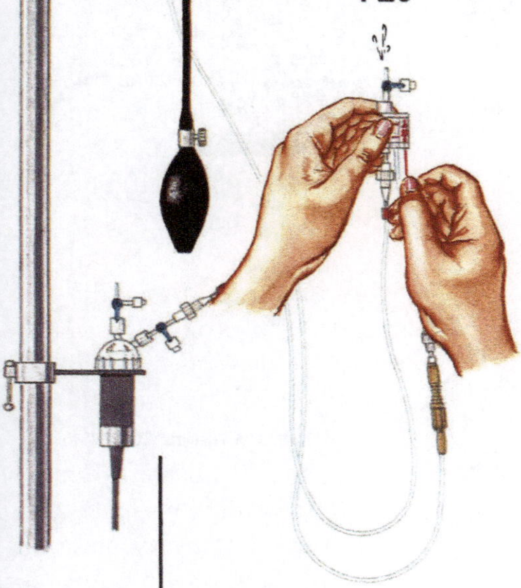

Verify stopcock positions and **Return to step F 12**

NO

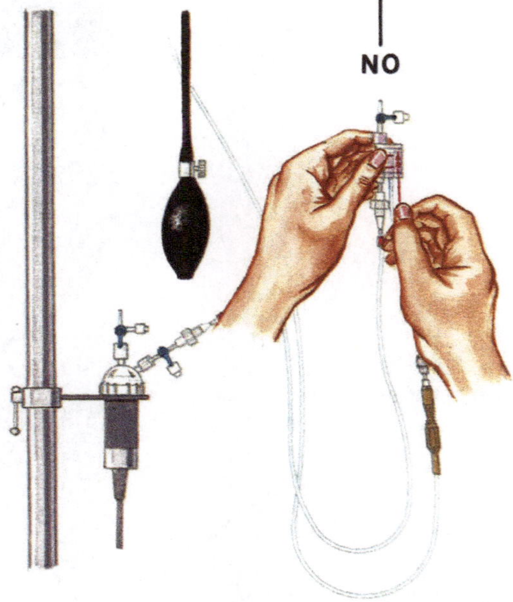

Continue

Step F15. Release Intraflo valve. Maintain sterility of patient tip connection.

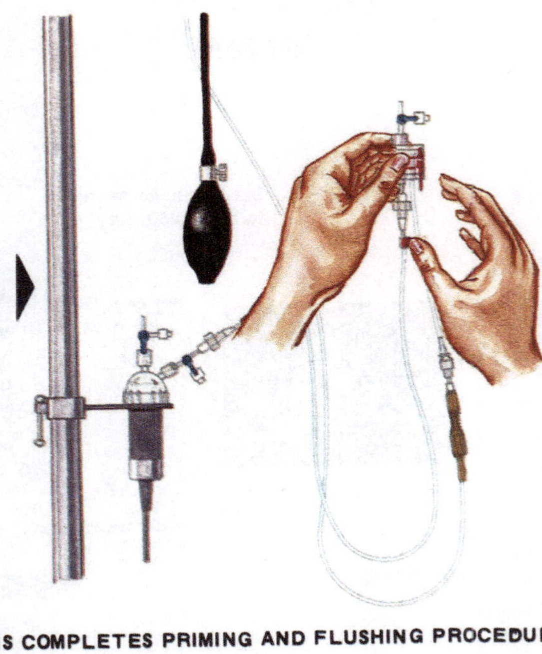

THIS COMPLETES PRIMING AND FLUSHING PROCEDURE

ZERO AND CALIBRATION PROCEDURE: MONITOR PREPARATION

Switch power "ON". The traces appear on the screen.

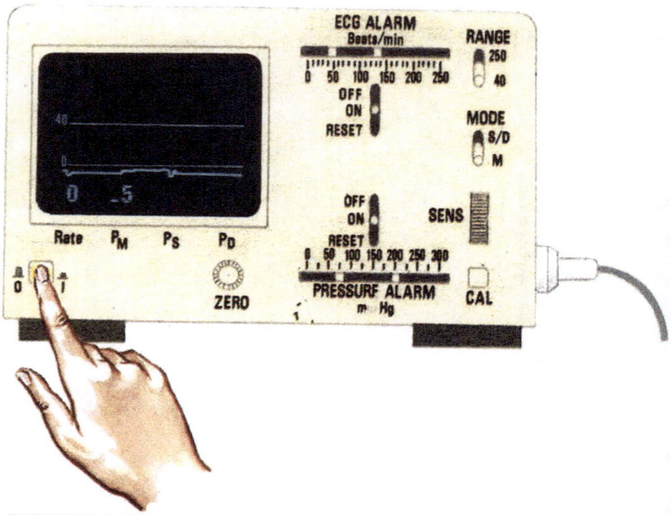

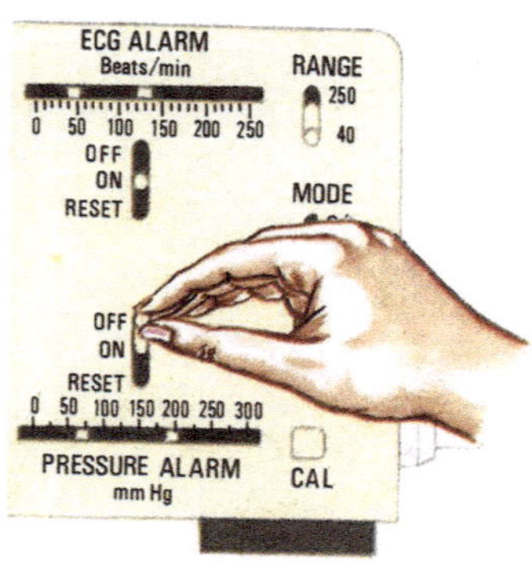

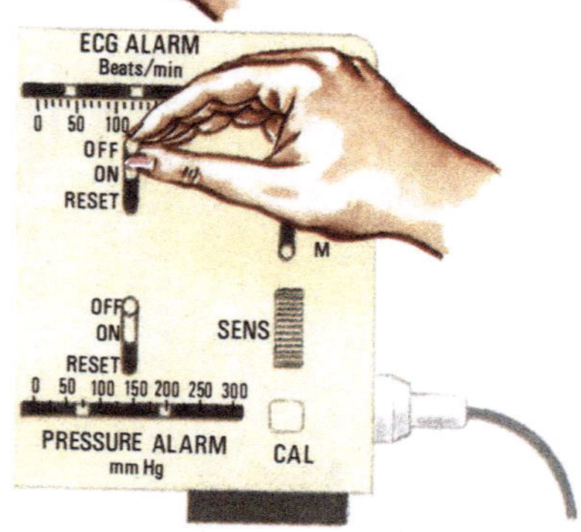

Turn the alarms "OFF".

Set the function switch to systolic.

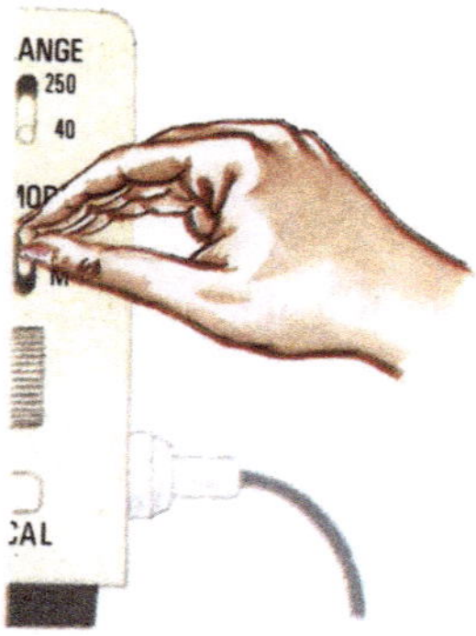

Set the range switch to high (250 mmHg)

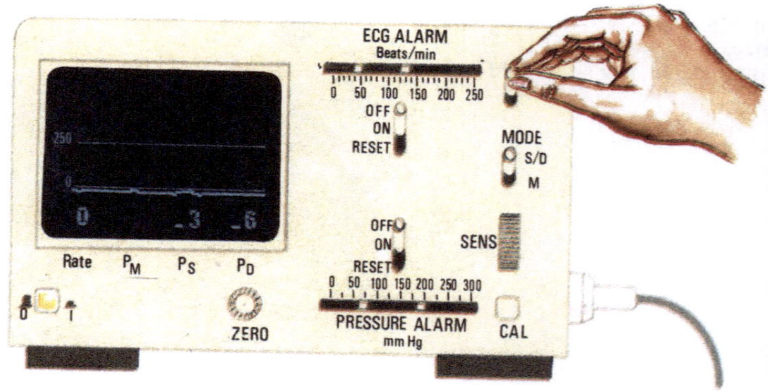

ZERO AND CALIBRATION PROCEDURE:
TRANSDUCER LEVELING

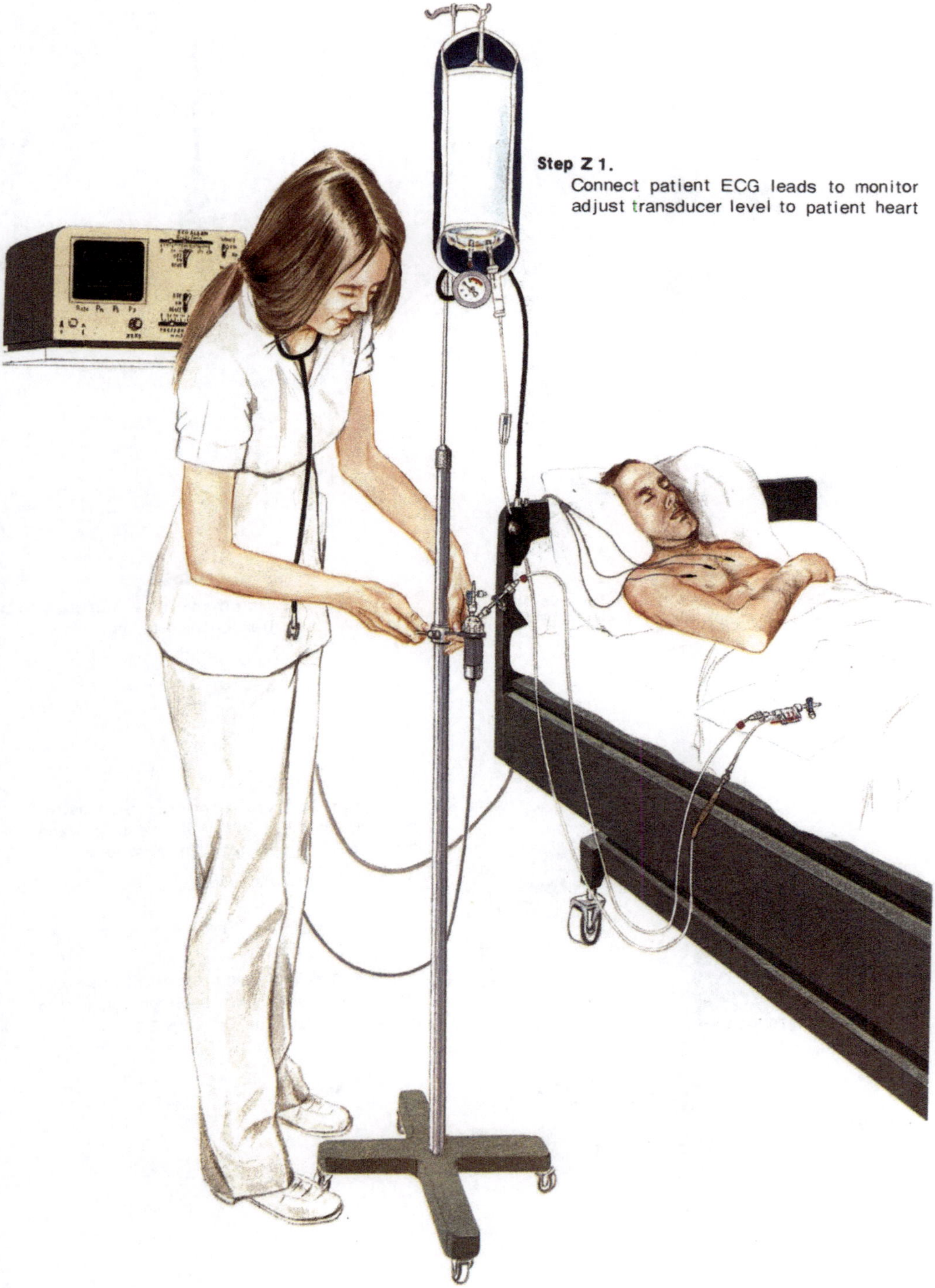

Step Z 1.
Connect patient ECG leads to monitor
adjust transducer level to patient heart

ZERO AND CALIBRATION PROCEDURE: ZEROING TRANSDUCER VS. ATMOSPHERE

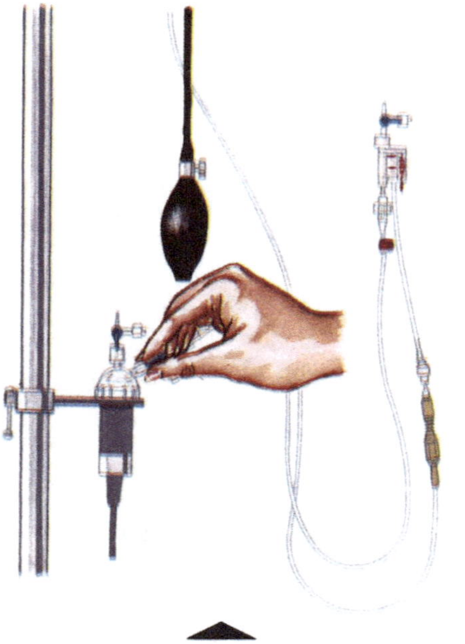

Step Z 2. Position the stopcock on the side of the transducer dome closed (OFF) to the dome.

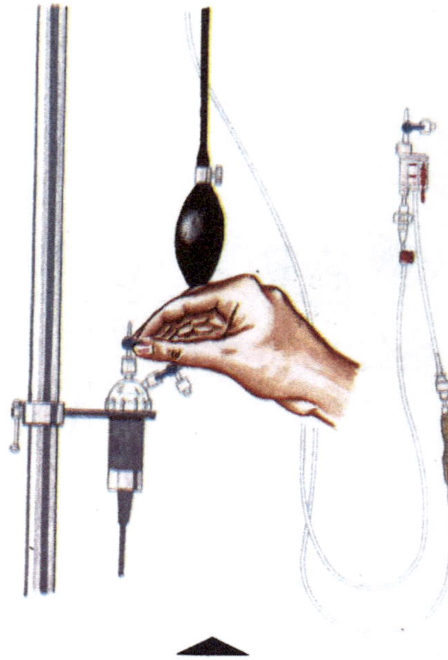

Step Z 3 Turn the vertical stopcock on the transducer dome open to air.

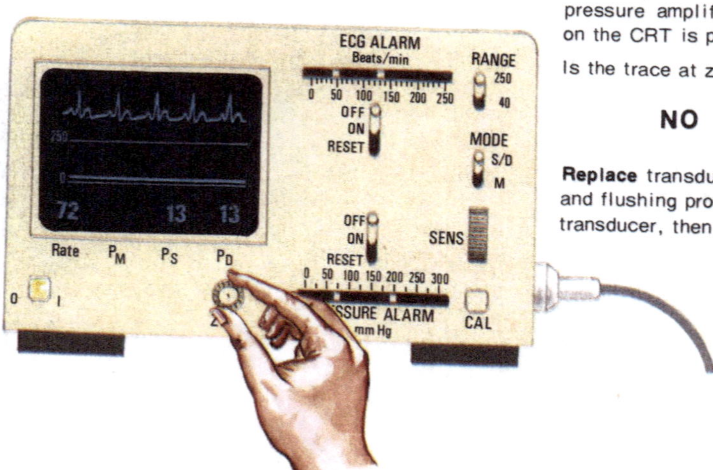

Step Z 4. Turn or press "zero" control on the monitor pressure amplifier until the pressure trace on the CRT is positioned at zero level.

Is the trace at zero level?

NO

Replace transducer and repeat all assembly and flushing procedure sections concerning transducer, then start at **step Z 1.**

ZERO AND CALIBRATION PROCEDURE: MONITOR VERIFICATION AND CALIBRATION

Plate Pl. 14

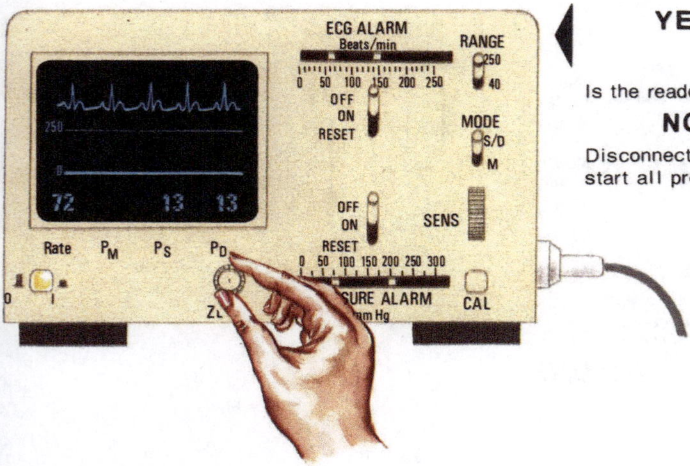

Step Z 5. Is the trace at zero level?

YES ⟶ **Continue**

Is the readout 0±1 mmHg?

NO

Disconnect, rechek or repair the monitor, then start all preparatory procedures again.

Step Z 6.

Is readout 0±1 mmHg?

YES

↓

Continue

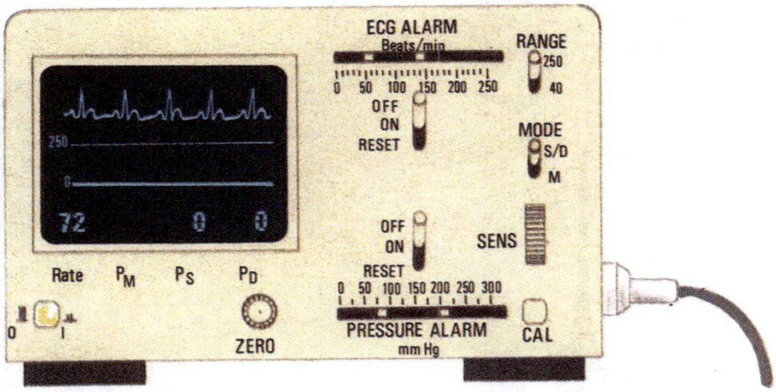

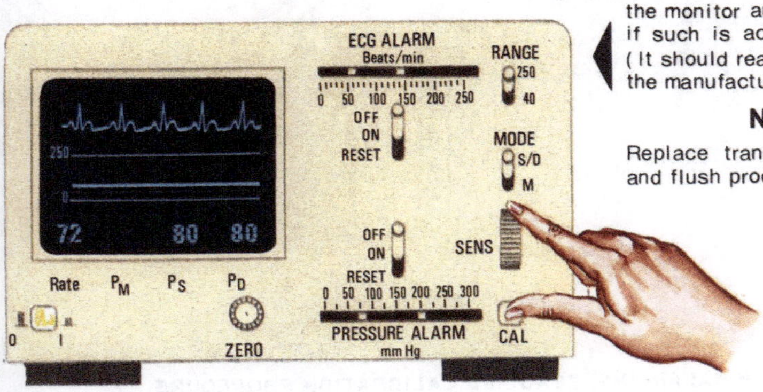

Step Z 7. Activate and hold the CALIBRATION switch on the monitor and adjust sensibility (gain) control if such is accessible. Is the readout correct? (It should read a precalibrated value stated by the manufacturer, e.g., 100 mmHg.)

NO

Replace transducer then repeat all assembly and flush procedures then restart at **Step Z 1.**

ZERO AND CALIBRATION PROCEDURE (CONTINUED)

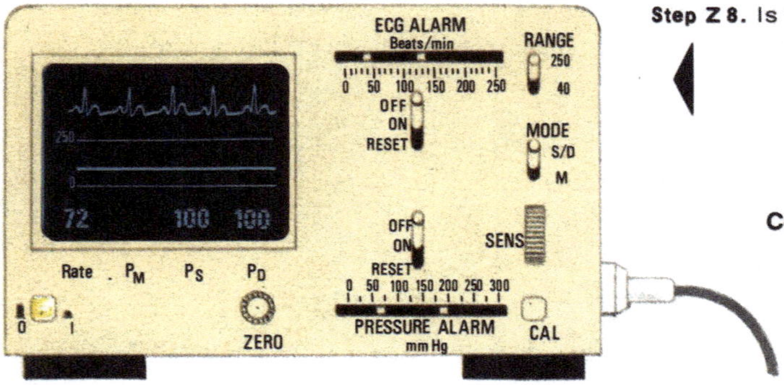

Step Z 8. Is the readout correct?

YES

Continue

Step Z 9.

Reposition stopcock valves to be ready for the monitoring. This maens closing off the vertical stopcock on the transducer dome to air.

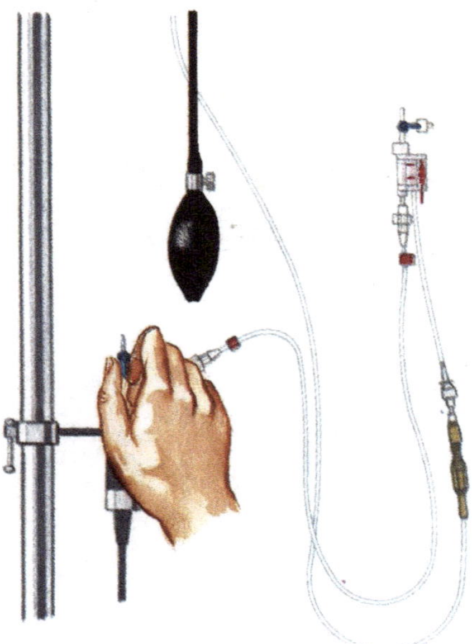

Step Z 10.

Open the transducer dome side stopcock to pressure tubing.

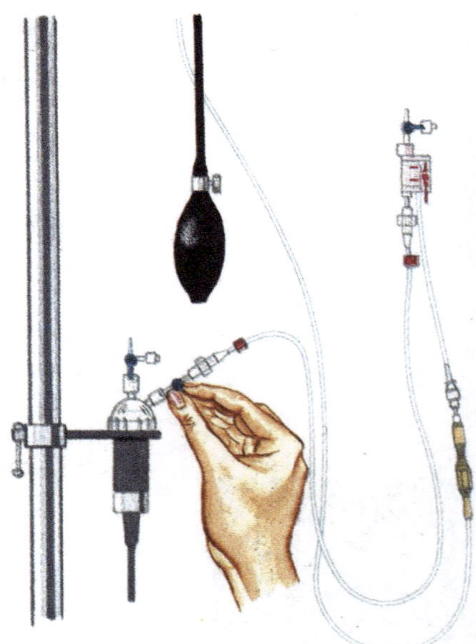

THIS CONCLUDES THE BALANCING, ZERO AND CALIBRATION PROCEDURE.

Step T 1. Turn the stopcock on the side of the transducer dome to be closed to the pressure tubing.

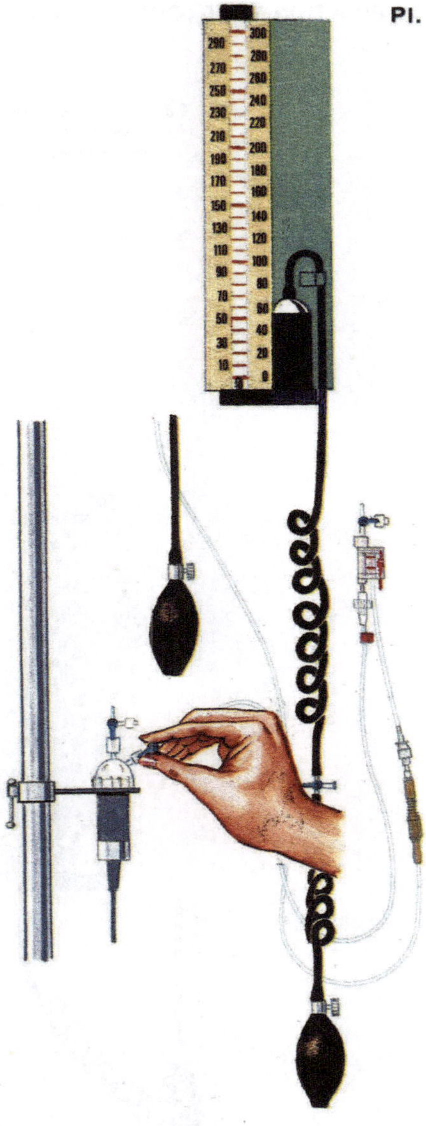

Step T 2.

Connect the manometer tubing via stopcock in T-connector arrangement to the vertical stopcock on the transducer dome. Note the deliberate absence of a sphygmomanometer cuff.

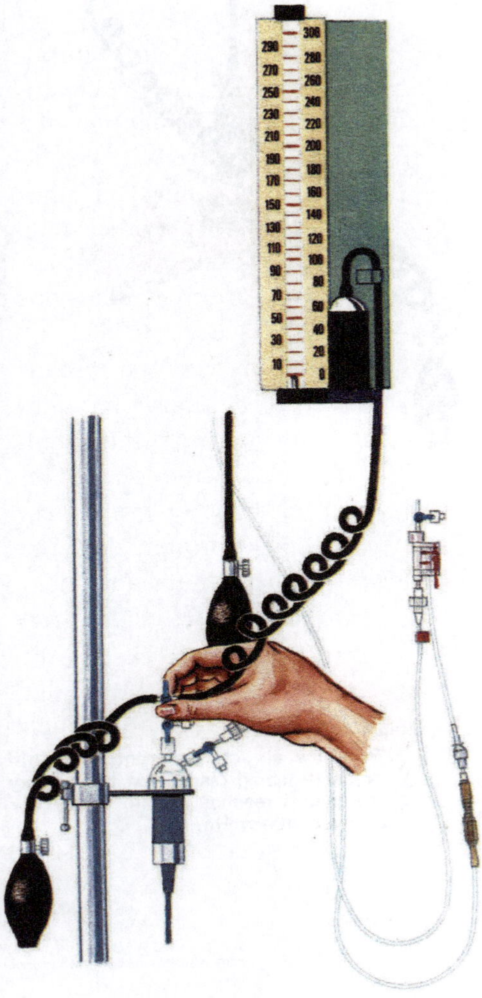

Step T 3. Open transducer dome vertical stopcock to the T-connector and the sphygmomanometer tubing.

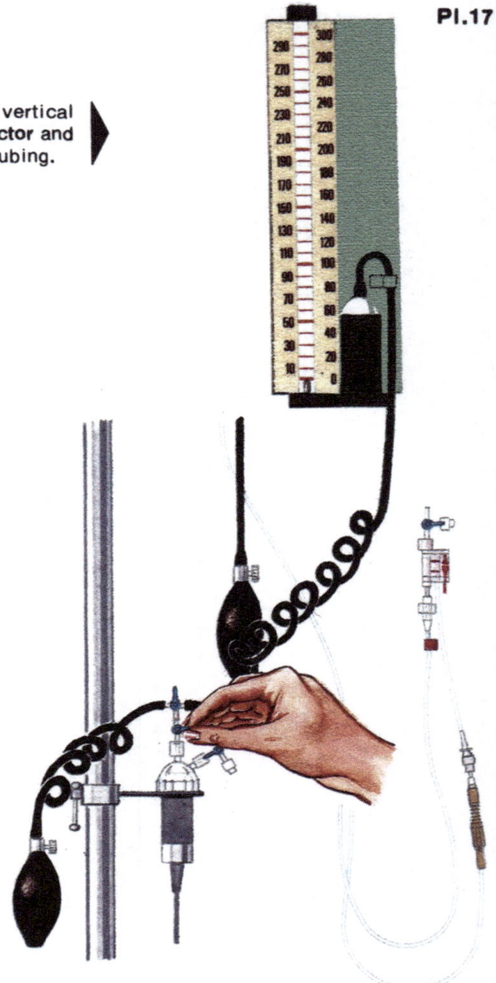

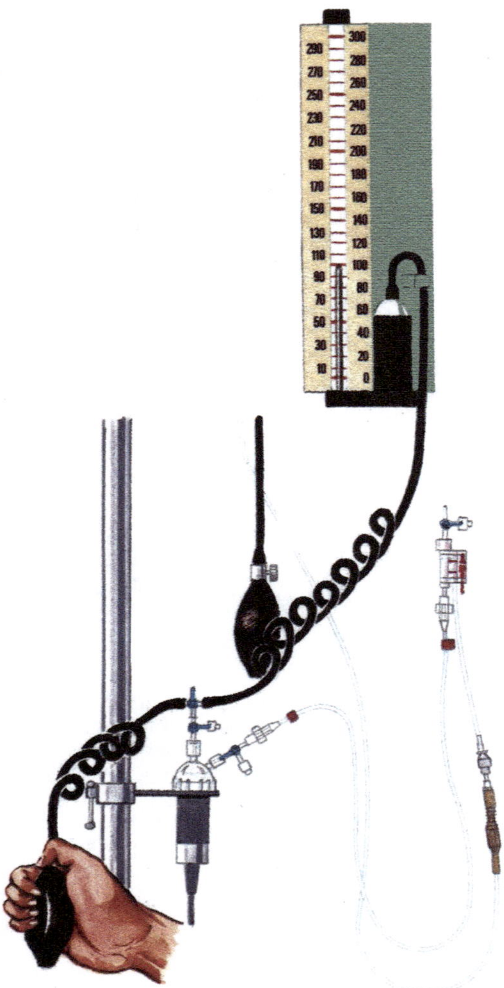

Step T 4.

Pump the air into the manometer until pressure tubing readout on the mercury the column reaches certain height, for example, 100 mmHg.

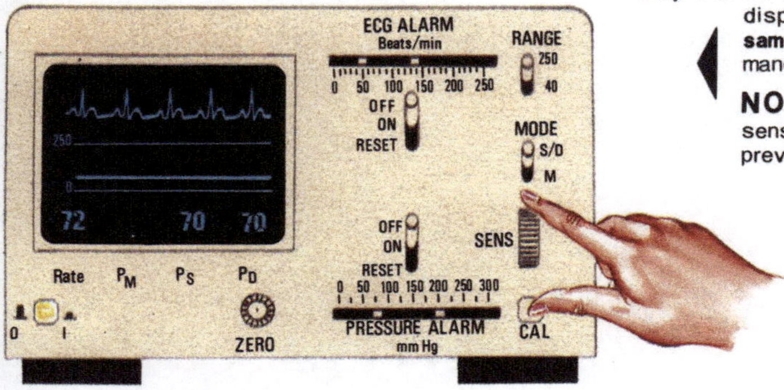

Step T 5. Do the trace on the CRT and numerical display on the monitor indicate the **same** (± 2%) pressure as the mercury manometer.

NO ⟶ Adjust the monitor sensitivy (gain) or check zero using previously described procedures.

YES

↓

Continue

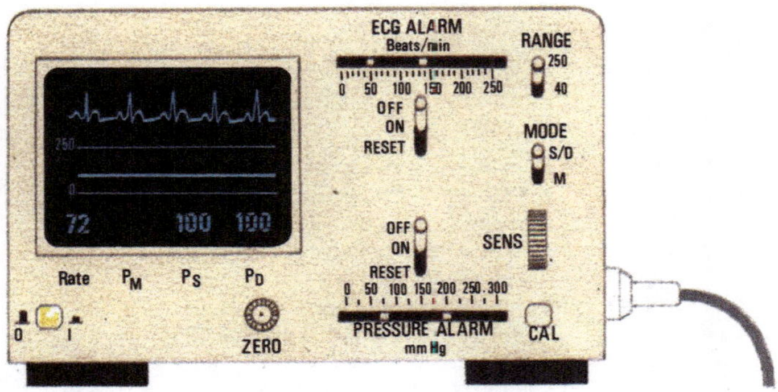

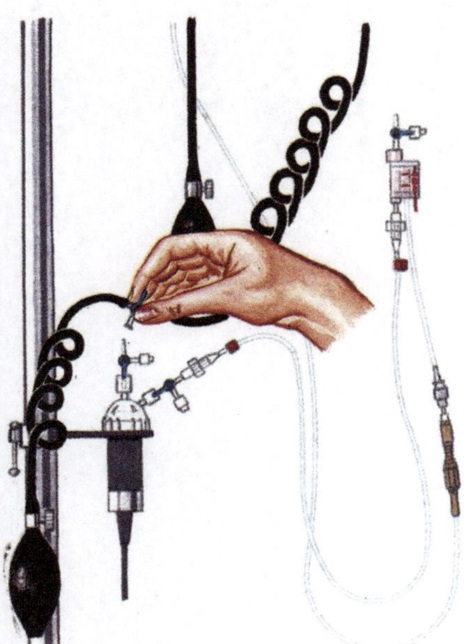

Step T6.

Bleed air from the mercury manometer, turn OFF to T-connector the vertical stopcock on the transducer dome and disconnect the T-connector.

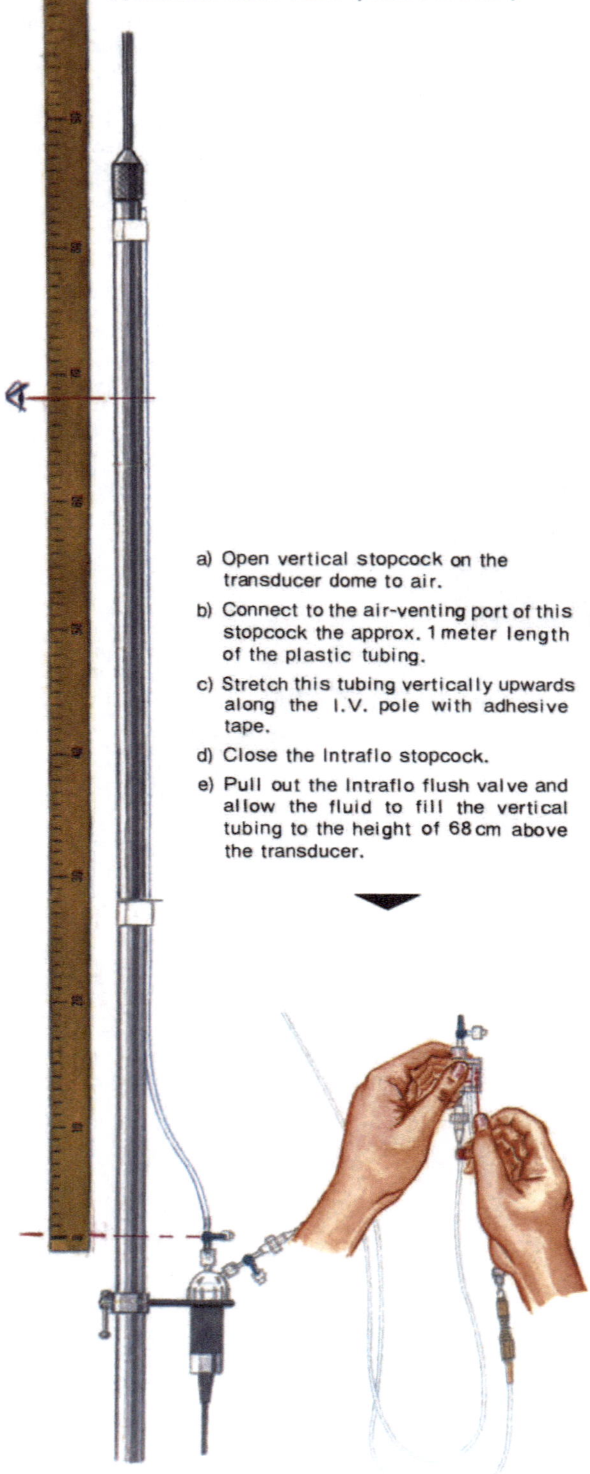

a) Open vertical stopcock on the transducer dome to air.
b) Connect to the air-venting port of this stopcock the approx. 1 meter length of the plastic tubing.
c) Stretch this tubing vertically upwards along the I.V. pole with adhesive tape.
d) Close the Intraflo stopcock.
e) Pull out the Intraflo flush valve and allow the fluid to fill the vertical tubing to the height of 68 cm above the transducer.

Step T 7.

Turn the stopcock on the side of the dome open to pressure line to resume monitoring.

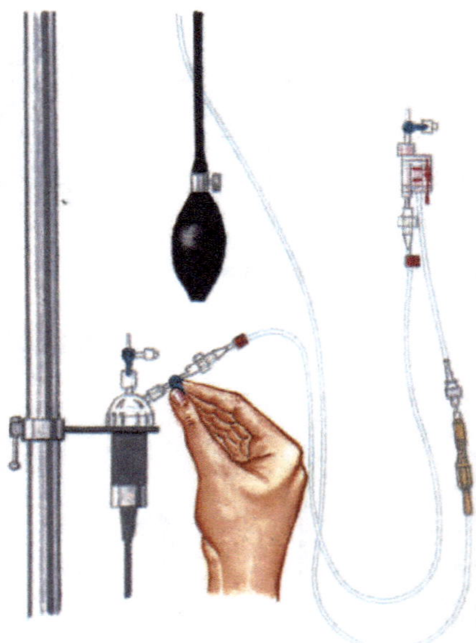

IX - DIRECT ARTERIAL PRESSURE MONITORING

The importance and clinical implifications of arterial pressure monitoring may be well illustrated by citing two examples described by Schroeder and Daily [1]:

Example I: A 38 year-old man with a massive diaphragmatic myocardial infarction was admitted to the coronary care unit. Four hours after admission he was confused, cool, clammy and had no urinary output. Cuff blood pressure was 70/50 mmHg. He was given norepinephrine and there was some improvement in his mental status and urinary output; however, a palpable radial artery pressure was estimated at only 70 mmHg. An intra-arterial brachial artery catheter was placed in the right arm. The actual pressure was 120/85 mmHg. The rate of norepinephrine administration therefore was decreased; his improvement was maintained and was reflected in an incerease in urinary output. Without the accurate intra-arterial pressure measurement, it would have been quite easy to further increase the norepinephrine, causing a continued rise in blood pressure due to excessive vasoconstriction, resulting in increased cardiac work and a potentially detrimental outcome.

Example II: A 72 year-old woman developed thrombophlebitis and had a massive pulmonary embolism on hospital day 2. Although her urinary outpout was apparently normal and femoral pulses were fair to good, a cuff blood pressure was not obtainable. An intra-arterial needle in the radial artery demonstrated a blood pressure of 105/90 mmHg. She was treated conservatively, and results were good.

9.1. Preparation of materials

Before starting the arterial monitoring procedure all the preparations described in Chapter 8 should be completed. The I.V. pole with flush system and transducer should be placed on the same side of the patient as the site of insertion. The key materials for arterial line insertion are illustrated on Plate 20.

Other auxilary materials not shown on the plate:

— armboard
— sterile gauze pads
— restraint
— 1% xylocaine & 3 cc syring ≠ 25 gauge needle
— sterile alcohol wipe
— waterproof pad
— alcohol, iodine, acetone, benzoin in convenient bottles
— adhesive tape
— sterile 4·0 silk suture on straight cutting needle
— pair of sterile gloves
— blood pressure cuff with pump

DIRECT ARTERIAL PRESSURE MONITORING
Catheter insertion technique into radial artery

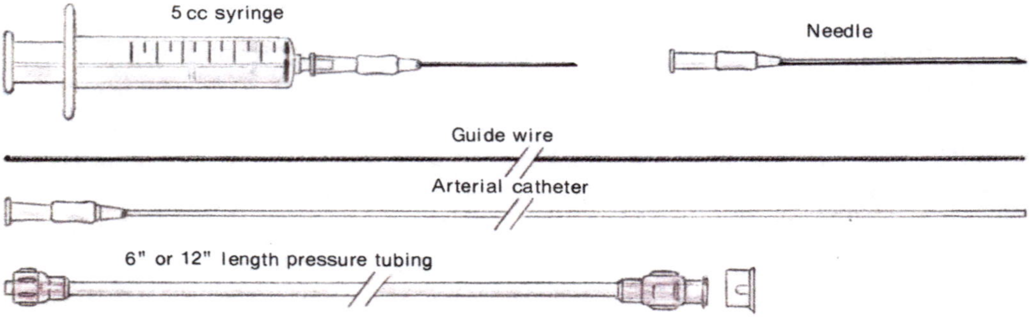

Step C 1 to C 4
(*see* **texte p.**)

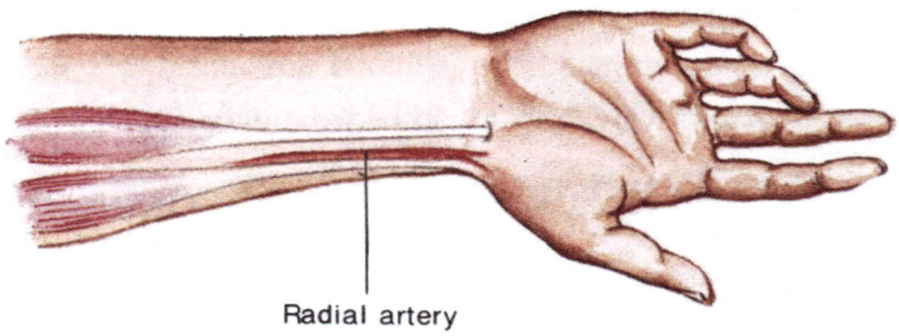

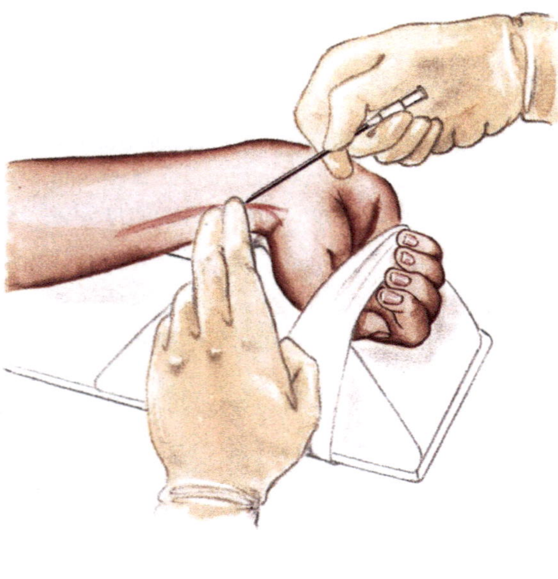

Step C 5 Insert the hypodermic gauge 18 sterile needle into the artery.

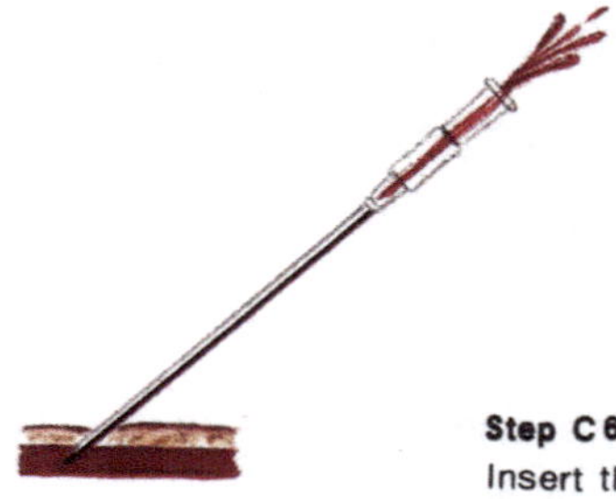

Step C 6
Insert the guide wire.

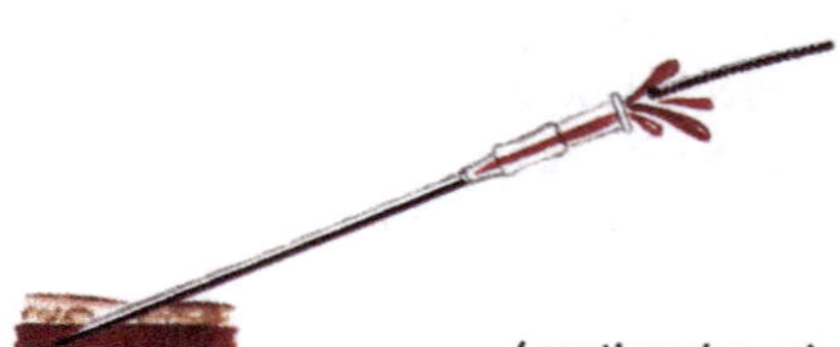

(continued on pl. 21)

9.2. Insertion sites

The commonly used sites for the introduction of arterial catheter are: radial, brachial and femoral arteries. They are illustrated on Fig. 13. Each site has some advantages and drawbacks concerning the ease of catheter-insertion and maintenance. In the first place the radial artery insertion is recommended for ease of maintenance. The palpation and location of insertion site is quite easy but the catheter-insertion into the radial artery is more difficult than in other sites due to its smaller size. The larger calibre of the femoral artery makes it the easiest to puncture and catheterize, but it is the most difficult site for continuous monitoring due to the difficulty in controlling active bleeding or oozing at the insertion site.

The complexity of brachial arterial catheterization lies between that of femoral and radial approaches.

In summary then, the site selection for arterial catheter insertion is a compromise between the ease of insertion versus the ease and safety of long-term maintenance. The radial artery is recommended as the site of choice for the sake of ease of maintenance and relative safety.

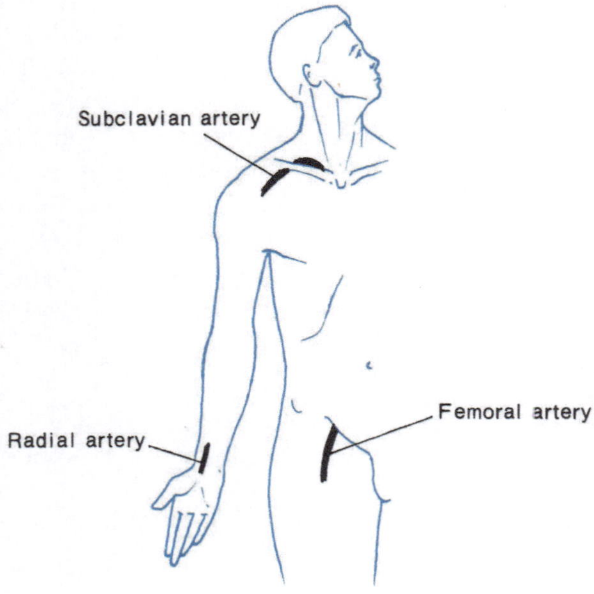

Fig. 13 - Arterial sites

9.3. Testing radial artery site

Before catheterizing the radial artery it is advisable to perform Allen's test to ensure adequate blood supply to the patient's hand if the artery should become occluded (thrombosed). To perform this test, occlude both the radial and ulnar arteries at the wrist after the hand has been held above the head and exercised. Then lower the hand and release the ulnar artery only. The hand should become pink if the blood supply is adequate. If this is not the case select an alternative insertion site.

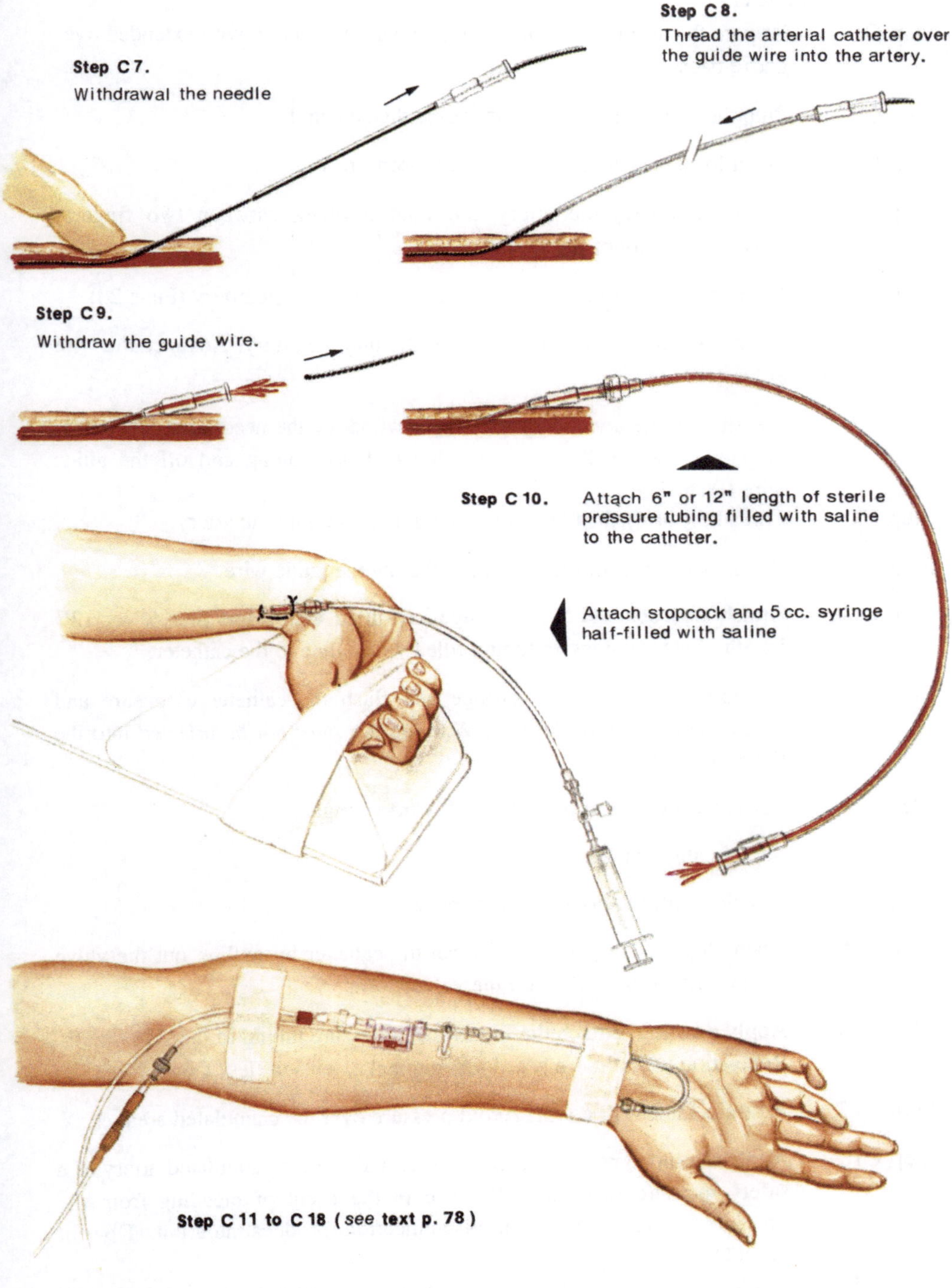
Step C 7.
Withdrawal the needle
Step C 8.
Thread the arterial catheter over the guide wire into the artery.
Step C 9.
Withdraw the guide wire.
Step C 10.
Attach 6" or 12" length of sterile pressure tubing filled with saline to the catheter.
Attach stopcock and 5 cc. syringe half-filled with saline
Step C 11 to C 18 (*see* **text p. 78**)

9.4. Insertion technique (Seldinger)

The step-by-step procedure as follows is recommended: (''C'' denotes catheter).

Step C1. — Prepare the arm by securing it to the board with wrist hyperextended over gauze pads.

Step C2. — Prep. the skin on the wrist with iodine then alcohol.

Step C3. — Inject local anesthetic into intended insertion site.

Step C4. — Locate (palpate) the artery and hold it down between two fingers. Preserve sterility of the site.

Step C5. — Insert the hypodermic gauge 18 sterile needle into the artery (Plate 20).

Step C6. — Insert the guide wire through the needle into the artery. Advance the wire at least 10 cm.

Step C7. — Pressing on the artery with the finger withdraw the needle but leave wire in place. The needle should be threaded back along and off the guide wire (Plate 21).

Step C8. — Thread the arterial catheter over the guide wire into the artery.

Step C9. — When catheter is all the way in, withdraw the guide wire.

Step C10. — Attach stopcock and 5 cc. syringe half-filled with saline plus 6'' or 12'' length of sterile pressure tubing filled with saline to the catheter.

Step C11. — Aspirate blood with the syringe and flush the catheter to ensure and check the patency of the line. Warning: air *must not be injected* into the tubing or catheter.

Step C12. — Turn stopcock off to patient and discard syringe.

Step C13. — Suture catheter to skin.

Step C14. — Attach Intraflo to arterial line stopcock.

Step C15. — Open stopcock to patient and flush the catheter by pulling out the valve on the Intraflo unit. Release the valve.

Step C16. — Apply dressing. Attach the Intraflo and pressure tubing to the skin. Reposition wrist on armboard for minimal extension (less than 30°).

Step C17. — Restrain catheterized arm. Avoid pressure over the cannulated area.

Step C18. — Apply the blood pressure cuff to the arm above the cannulated artery as a safety measure to occlude the arm in the event of bleeding from the pressure system, accidental disconnection or decannulation. Do not inflate the cuff.

This concludes the description of the recommended catheter insertion technique into radial artery.

9.5. Normal arterial pressure tracing

The commonly observed normal brachial or radial artery pressure tracing shows a rapid upstroke, systolic peak value of above 120 mmHg, followed by the decline with the notch (dichrotic) down to minimum diastolic value of approx. 70 mmHg, followed by the next systolic upstroke

(Fig. 14).

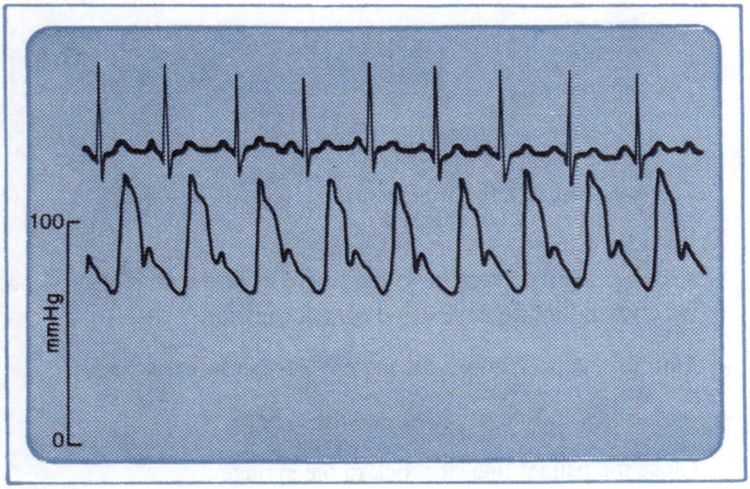

Fig. 14 - Radial artery pressure tracing in a normal subject

9.6. Damped tracing and what to do about it

If the arterial pressure tracing becomes flattened and appears smoothed it may indicate *damping* due to a clot formation or an air bubble in the system (Fig. 15).

To remedy the situation there are two consecutive actions:

1. The possible clot in the catheter should be removed.
2. The pressure tubing-transducer system should be flushed.

The recommended clot and air removal technique is: ("D" denotes *damped* tracing).

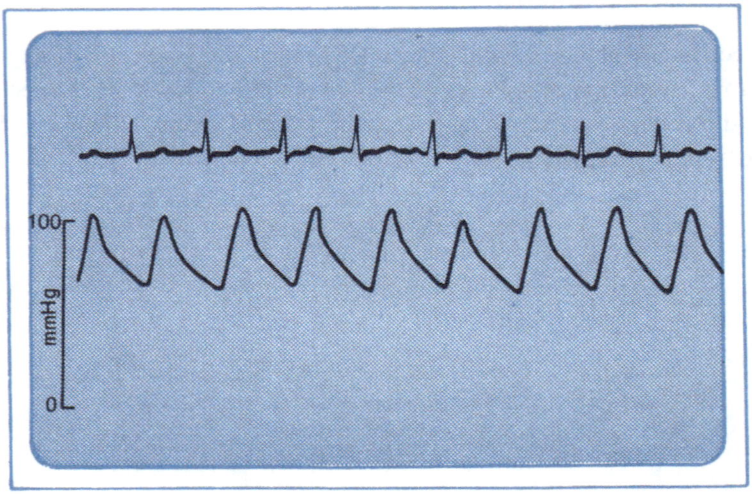

Fig. 15 - Damped arterial pressure tracing due to a clot or air in the catheter

Step D1. — Attach 5 to 10 cc syringe to the side port of the three-way stopcock which is between Intraflo device and patient catheter.

Step D2. — Turn this stopcock open the patient catheter to the syringe.

Step D3. — *Withdraw* ca. 5 ml of blood into the syringe.

Step D4. — Close the patient line stopcock to the syringe.

Step D5. — Discard the syringe.

Step D6. — Pull out the flush valve on the Intraflo system and release it after a few seconds. Flush the patient catheter. Allow for approx. 20 cc of a flushing fluid to be infused into patient.

Step D7. — Flush the possible air bubble from pressure tubing and transducer dome system using Steps F1 through F11 from Chapter 8.

Step D8. — Reread the pressure tracing.

If the damped trace still persists on the screen, there might be medical reason for the slow upstroke and a virtual disappearance of a dichrotic notch. Damped-appearing trace may be seen in patients with severe valvular aortic stenosis, marked peripheral vasoconstriction or conditions of circulatory collapse.

9.7. Maintenance of catheter patency

The most effective way of catheter patency maintenance is the continuous flush using the Intraflo system as described in Chapter 6. It should be supervised however and frequently checked for proper operation (e.g. proper drip rate of ca 3 cc/hour in the

IV chamber, infusion bag cuff pressure of approx. 300 mmHg, etc.). Even with the continuous flush system, thrombus formation almost invariably occurs, to at least a small degree. To prevent the clot or miniclots from entering the vascular system withdraw some blood through the catheter and flush the system periodically (e.g. every four hours), as described in steps D1 to D6.

9.8. Patient protection measures

It is important to keep the hand with the arterial line uncovered, so that it may be frequently and easily observed. This is to prevent prolonged (and possibly fatal) bleeding due to an inadvertant loose connection in the tubing system. The pulse distal to the arterial catheter should be checked every 2 hours for early detection of obstruction or thrombosis in the extremity.

The transducer dome and the tubing should be filled with flush fluid *all the time* and be free of air bubbles or blood. If blood does back up into the transducer for any reason, the whole tubing-dome-flush system should be disconnected from the patient and affected sections replaced. Before reconnection to the patient, the assembly and filling procedures (pp. 51 through 52) should be thoroughly implemented with special emphasis on maintaining the sterility of the system.

To prevent infection, all components which may come in contact via flush fluid with the patient's blood stream should be replaced periodically (recommended cycle: 48 hours). This includes: all stopcocks, all pressure tubing, Intraflo flush system, infusion fluid and IV set and the transducer dome (if disposable, presterilized dome is used). The entire transducer should be replaced when a non-disposable dome is used (without a sterile isolation barrier between the fluid-filled space and the transducer diaphragm).

9.9. Problems encountered with arterial catheters

— Hematoma at a puncture site may result from bleeding or oozing after withdrawal of the catheter. It could be prevented by maintaining firm pressure on the site during withdrawal and for 5 to 15 minutes after withdrawing the catheter.

— Decreased or absent pulse distal to the insertion site may be caused either by arterial spasm or thrombosis of artery. The former may be prevented by clean, non traumatic arterial puncture technique or treated by local injection of lidocaine. The latter is caused by mechanical trauma or obstruction to the artery. To minimize this risk use clean, well-experienced technique avoiding multiple punctures of the vessel for insertion. Check the the distal pulse after insertion and hourly thereafter. The treatment for this condition is arteriotomy and Fogarty catheterization both distally and proximally from the puncture site.

9.10. Left ventricular and aortic pressure

All the components and settings of the arterial pressure monitoring system are the same for the purpose of left ventricular pressure monitoring. To facilitate the entry to the heart, longer, stiffer and preformed catheters with guidewires are used. The introduction site is usually the left femoral artery and the catheter is advanced retrograde through the aorta with simultaneous electrocardiographic monitoring. During catheter passage through the aortic valve into the left ventricule, some ectopic beats usually occur due to mechanical stimulation of the heart muscle. The entry of the catheter tip into the left ventricle is confirmed by a marked change in the pressure tracing on a CRT. While the peak left ventricular systolic pressure in normal subjects remains the same as that in the root of the aorta, the diastolic pressure is very *low* — down to a few mmHg (Fig. 16).

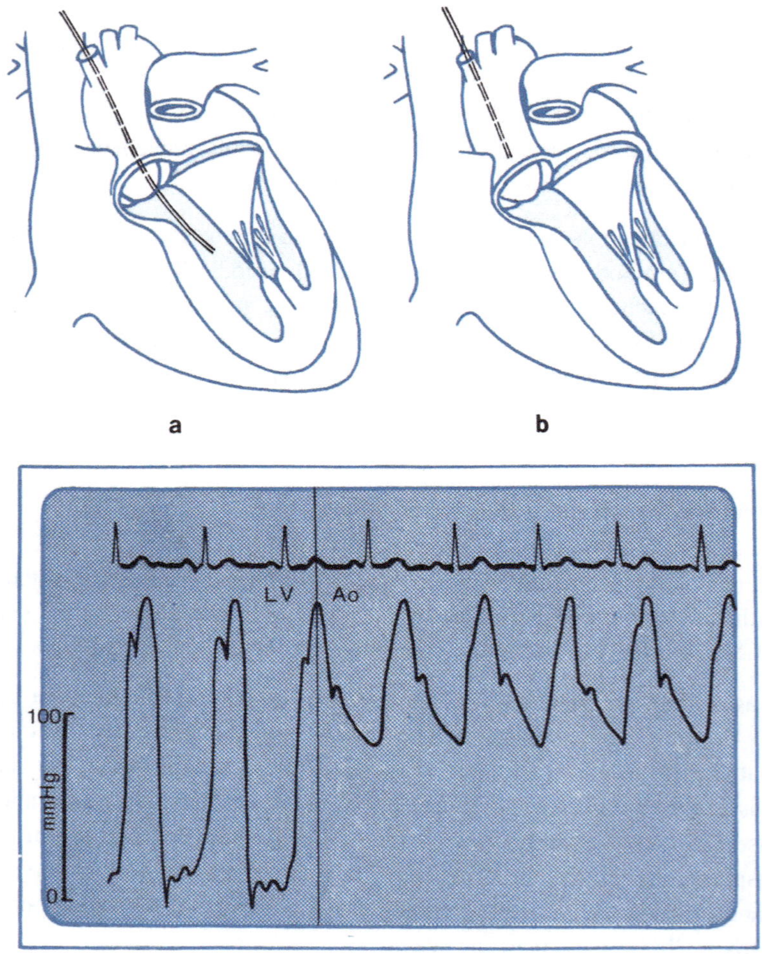

Fig. 16 • The change in pressure tracing as the catheter is pulled back from the left ventricle (LV) **(a)** to the aorta (Ao) **(b)**

Some of the clinical conditions which can be easily diagnosed by monitoring of left ventricular/aortic pressure include:

— Aortic stenosis resulting in a significantly lower peak systolic pressure in the aorta than in the left ventricle.

— Left ventricular failure resulting in elevated end diastolic pressure in LV (above 12 mmHg).

— Severe congestive heart failure resulting in profound LV dysfunction and pulsus alternans.

— Aortic insufficiency resulting in abnormally low diastolic pressure in the aorta (about 20 mmHg).

9.11. Guidelines for good monitoring

— Label arterial lines and infusion fluid.

— Keep infusion fluid pressurized above patient systolic pressure.

— Maintain catheter patency by continuous flush device.

— Frequently check all connections.

— Keep all connectors and puncture sites visible.

— Immobilize insertion site.

— Frequently check pulse and sensation distal to puncture site.

— Remedy damped tracing when necessary.

— Maintain transducer level with the heart.

— Verify zero and calibration from time to time.

— Test daily the monitoring system operation by measuring known pressure.

— Maintain flush fluid sterility at all times.

— Change system components every 48 hours to prevent infection.

— Keep constant vigilance for possible disconnections, bleeding and complications.

— Change dressing on the puncture site every 48 hours.

X - DIRECT CENTRAL VENOUS PRESSURE (CVP) MONITORING

CVP is most valuable in monitoring blood volume and adequacy of venous return in restrictive and constrictive disorders of the right heart. It is particularly helpful after surgery, during active bleeding or in assessing dehydration. Also, in constrictive lung disease, pulmonary edema and left heart failure it is a valuable guide for the regulation of fluid balance.

The CVP pressure is measured with the catheter tip in the midsuperior vena cava and it reflects the blood pressure in the right atrium. As this pressure corresponds to the *volume* of blood there it gives some indication of other important variables as cardiac output and arterial pressure. If the volume of returning blood decreases so does the CVP. In general, a pressure below 5 cmH_2O (= 3·7 mmHg) indicates a need for additional fluid volume to be given to the patient. This additional volume will cause an increase in CVP and will contribute to an increase in cardiac output and arterial pressure.

Although the CVP will eventually reflect left-sided heart failure or other severe abnormalities, the timing and sequence of the events are not predictable. Therefore, there is less value in CVP monitoring of patients with rapidly changing cardiovascular status.

10.1. Insertion sites

The most frequently used sites are large veins in the antecubital fossa namely the medial basilic. The external or internal jugular as well as subclavian veins may also be used.

The neck region sites are less comfortable for the patient but are best suited for longterm monitoring due to the very low incidence of thrombophlebitis there. The risk of inadvertant pneumothorax must be taken into account when using a subclavian vein site.

10.2. Insertion techniques

A large bore needle attached to an empty syringe is advanced into the vein. The location of the tip in the lumen of the vein is confirmed by withdrawal of a small amount of blood by negative pressure in a syringe. The syringe is then disconnected and a catheter is pushed through the needle to the vein and advanced into the superior vena cava. The catheter should advance easily. If persistant resistance to advancement occurs, the needle with the catheter should be withdrawn and a new puncture made. After insertion, the needle should be taped and secured so that it cannot dislodge or cut the catheter.

The appropriate CVP catheter length should be selected in order to reach the superior vena cava from the insertion site. It should be measured by holding the protected catheter form the proposed insertion site to the sternal notch. The sterility of puncture side and of the length of catheter in contact with the blood stream must be maintained at all times.

The above technique applied for subclavian vein insertion is illustrated on Plates 22 and 23.

10.3. Methods of CVP measurement

The conditions for CVP measurement are similar to those for arterial pressure monitoring with the exception of a lower pressure readout range on the monitor switch and lower pressure over the infusìon pack (ca 150 mmHg). While monitoring CVP with a water column manometer (see fig. 17), the measurement will be obtained in mm of water (mmH_2O). The conversion into kP or mmHg is given in Table 1 page 20.

The simplicity and low price of systems for the measurement of CVP pressure with the water column manometer are main advantages. The drawbacks are: lack of automatic alarms and lack of the facility for recording. In advanced critical care installations electronic CVP monitoring is used for the above reasons. The *mean* pressure modality is usually displayed and monitored.

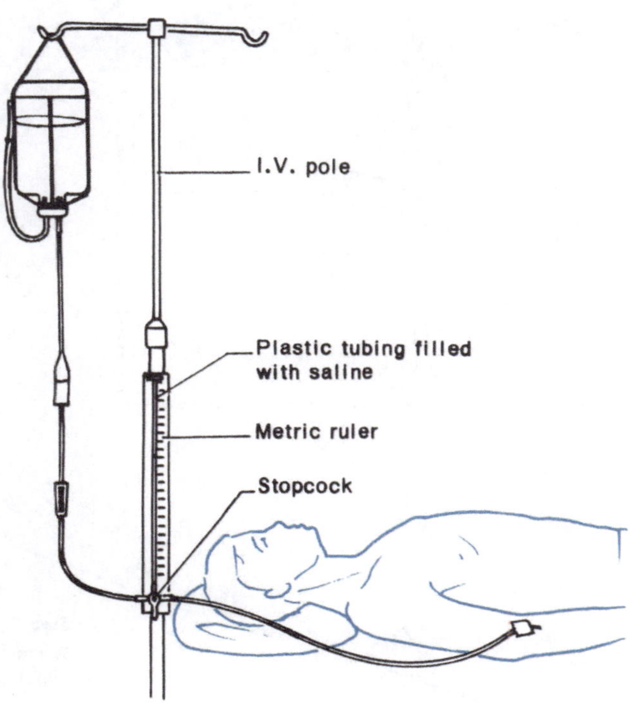

Fig. 17- Measuring of CVP with water column manometer

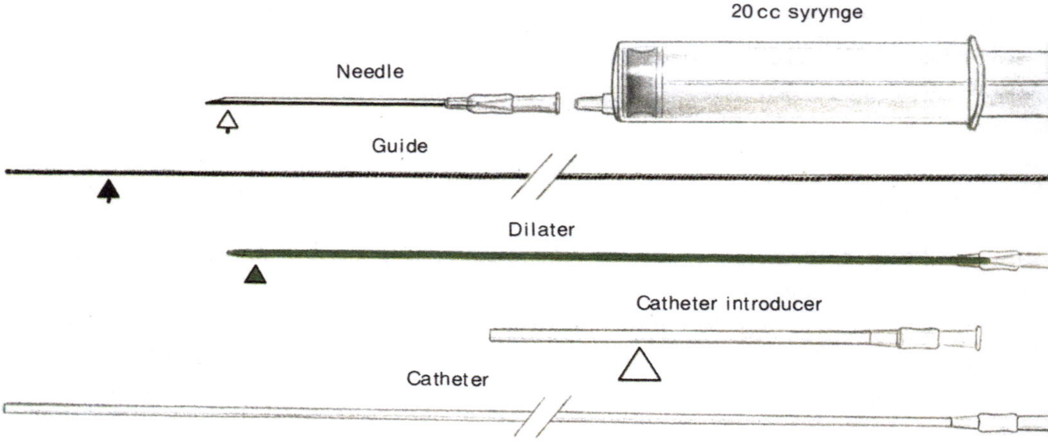

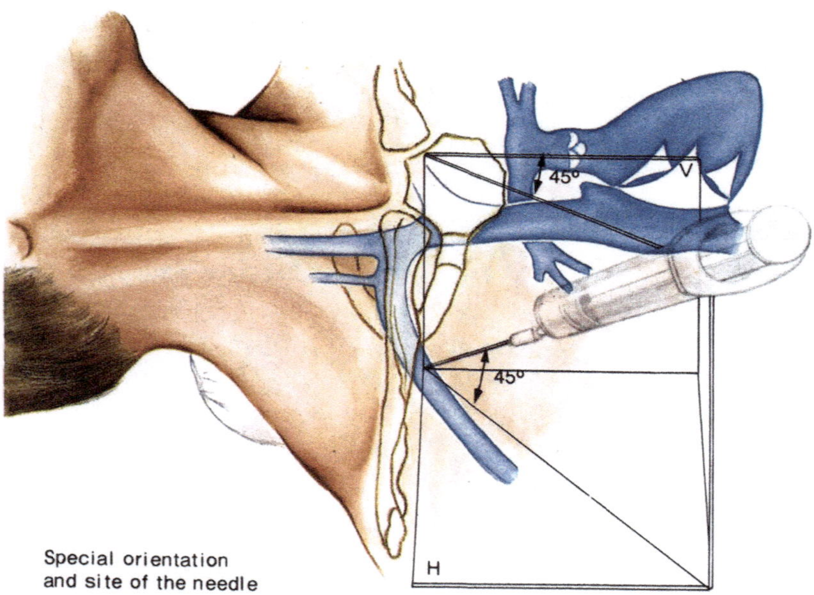

V = Vertical plane
H = Horizontal plane
(sternal plane)

Special orientation
and site of the needle

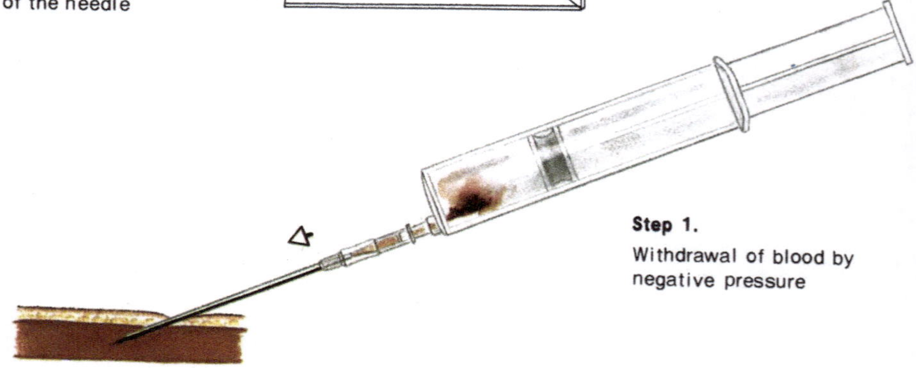

Step 1.
Withdrawal of blood by
negative pressure

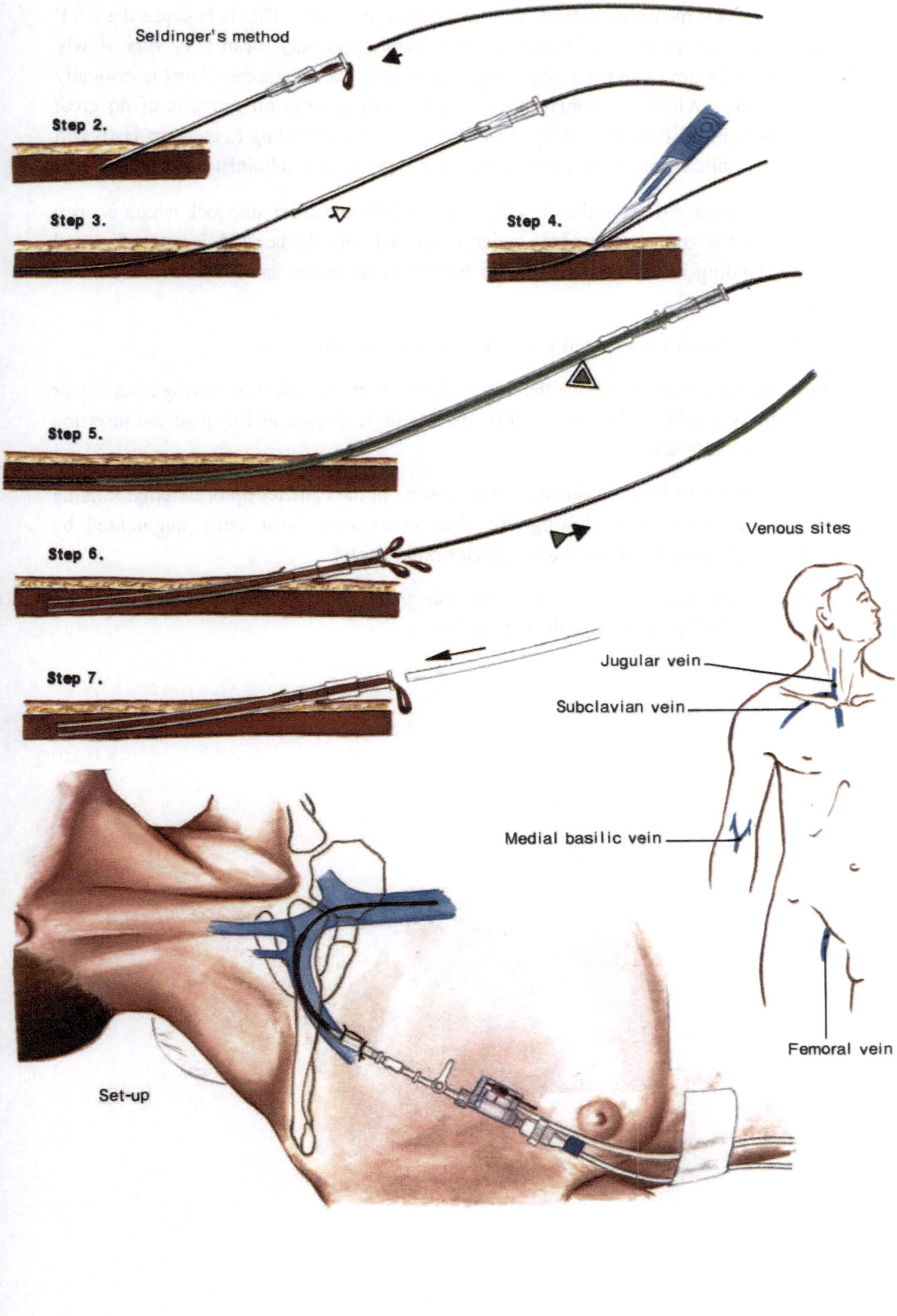
Seldinger's method
Step 2.
Step 3.
Step 4.
Step 5.
Step 6.
Step 7.
Venous sites
Jugular vein
Subclavian vein
Medial basilic vein
Femoral vein
Set-up

10.4. Problems with CVP measurements

The cather-tubing-transducer system configuration is not as important for the accuracy of CVP measurements as it is for arterial pressures. This is because the CVP signal to be reproduced is primarily static in nature and only mean (i.e. very slowly changing) levels are of interest. By contrast, the transducer reference *level* is critically important here. While a 3 mmHg error in measuring arterial pressures is of no great consequence, in CVP determination a similar error (corresponding to ca.4 cm H_2O) will have grave implications as such values are used to govern the administration of fluids.

It is emphasized again that it is the port (outlet) transducer stopcock which is open to air during the zeroing procedure which is leveled with the heart. Misconception and misunderstanding of the above will lead to significant errors and may seriously affect therapy.

Other problems associated with CVP catheters include:

— Pain and inflammation above the needle due to bacterial infection during insertion or to thrombophlebitis. To prevent this, use sterile technique and change the insertion site every 48 hours.

— Poor infusion of IV fluid due to partial clotting at the catheter tip or external kinking of tubing. To reduce clotting use slow continuous flush setup augmented by occasional blood withdrawal and catheter rapid flush.

— Catheter partially sheared during insertion or manipulation. To prevent *never* pull back the catheter on the needle and readvance.

XI - DIRECT PULMONARY ARTERY PRESSURE MONITORING

It has now been established (Rutherford et.al.[1]) that pulmonary artery pressure is an important parameter for continuous monitoring of left ventricular (LV) performance. A further factor for assessing LV performance is cardiac output. As stated before, cardiac output is the volume of blood ejected by the left ventricle in one minute (liters per minute). There are no instruments yet available for continuous measurement of blood flow. The presently-used methods for cardiac output determination are indirect, afford only sporadic measurements and are not simple. The good indicator for continuous assessment of cardiac output is left atrial pressure. This LA pressure is the same as the LV end-diastolic pressure which in turn relates to the stroke volume (Starling's Law). If we could insert and maintain a pressure monitoring catheter in the left atrium, continuous assessment of LV performance would be easier. It is posible to insert a retrograde arterial line all the way into the aorta and through the aortic valve into the left ventricle. However, the procedure requires a great degree of skill and the presence of a stiff catheter tip in the ventricle causes arrhythmias. Long-term monitoring of LV pressure is then not very feasible and presents the additional risk of catheter-introduced trauma or systemic emboli. An exciting medical advance in the 1970's was provided by the introduction of the balloon-tipped catheter by Swan, Ganz et.al.[3], to facilitate monitoring of the left atrial pressure. This is accomplished *without* placing the tip of the monitoring catheter into the left heart, thus avoiding the risks mentioned above. The catheter is placed in the pulmonary artery instead and when the balloon is temporarily inflated (so-called wedged), it seals off the catheter tip orifice from the pulmonary artery pressure. Thus the catheter tip ''sees'' the downstream pressure in the pulmonary capillaries which is a close and faithful representation of left ventricular filling pressure (i.e. LA pressure). The pulmonary vasculature serves the role of a fluid-filled passive extension of catheter tubing, and indeed terminates in the left atrium. The studies conducted by Lappas et.al.[4] on postsurgical patients compared direct LA pressures with pulmonary-capillary wedge pressures (PCWP). The difference was found to be so minimal (± 1 mmHg) that it was beyond the limits of clinical detection.

11.1. Preparation of materials (Swan-Ganz catheter).

The inflatable balloon on the tip of the Swan-Ganz catheter (Pl. 24,) serves four purposes. First, as the balloon is filled with air, it *floats* with the blood stream. Second, as the catheter is inserted into the vein, the balloon *directs* it toward the right heart and thence into pulmonary arteries. Third, the balloon provide a ''cushion'' preventing the catheter tip from impinging upon cardiac tissues which are susceptible to arrhythmias if mechanically irritated. Fourth, the balloon wedges the catheter into a pulmonary artery branch and isolates the catheter orifice from the pulmonary arterial pressure pulse.

The key materials in addition to the Swan-Ganz catheter are identical to those used for CVP monitoring (Plate 22).

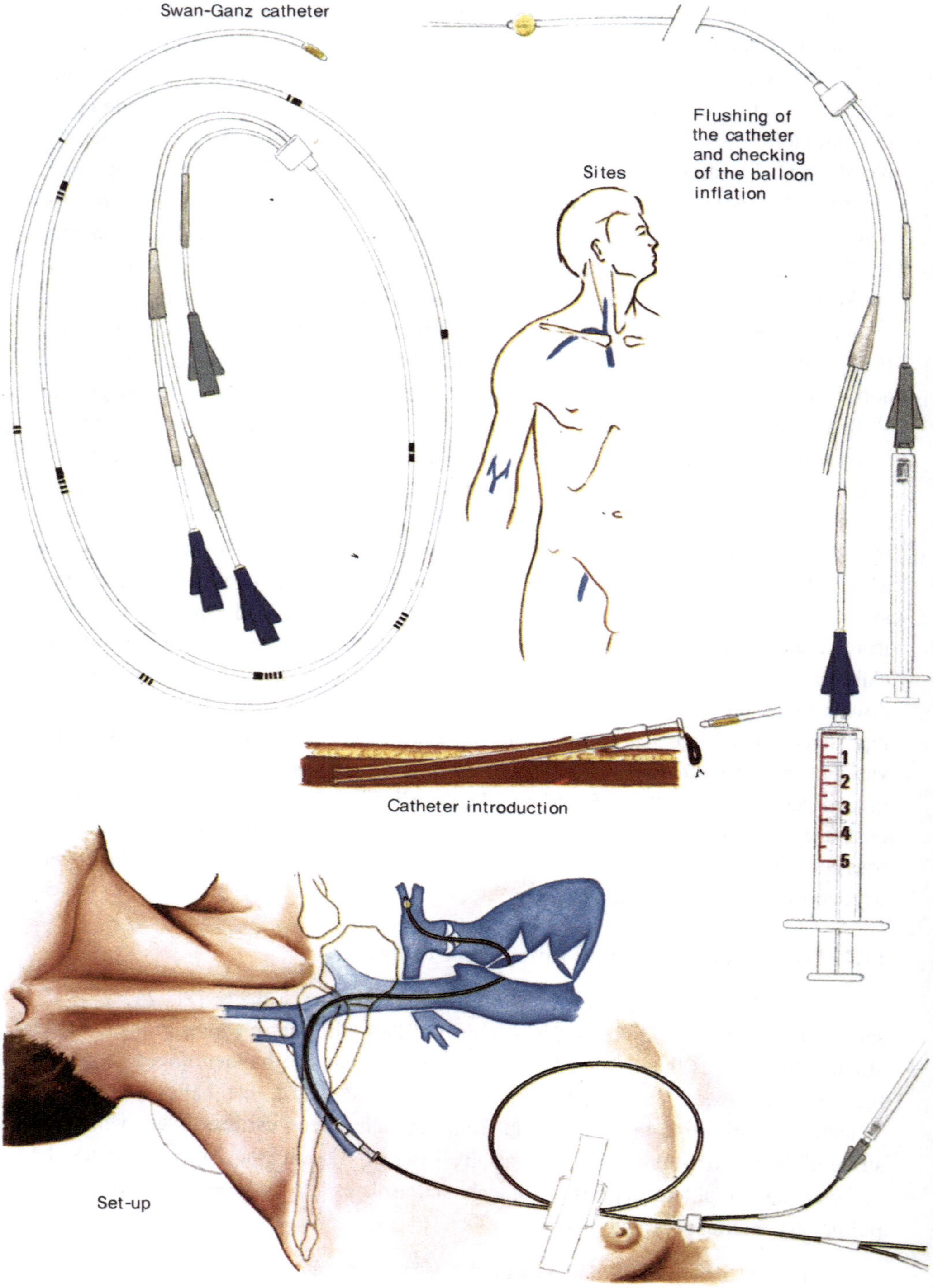
Swan-Ganz catheter
Sites
Flushing of the catheter and checking of the balloon inflation
1
2
3
4
5
Catheter introduction
Set-up

11.2. Insertion sites and technique

The balloon-tipped catheter may be inserted percutaneously, usually in the antecubital fossa with a needle, guide wire and catheter introducer. The introduction technique is so easy that it may be accomplished without prior catheterization laboratory experience and without the aid of fluoroscopy. It can be also inserted in the subclavian vein (Plate 22, 23). During insertion, the balloon is completely deflated until it fully enters the lumen of the vein. Advance the catheter (previously flushed and connected to a ready monitoring system — see Procedures, Chapter 8) toward the thorax. *Partially* inflate the balloon with air when the tip of the catheter reaches the shoulder level. This partially inflated balloon will float while the catheter is advanced downstream to the superior vena cava and the right atrium. Once the catheter tip reaches the atrium, which is confirmed by the tracing on the screen (Fig.18a), inflate

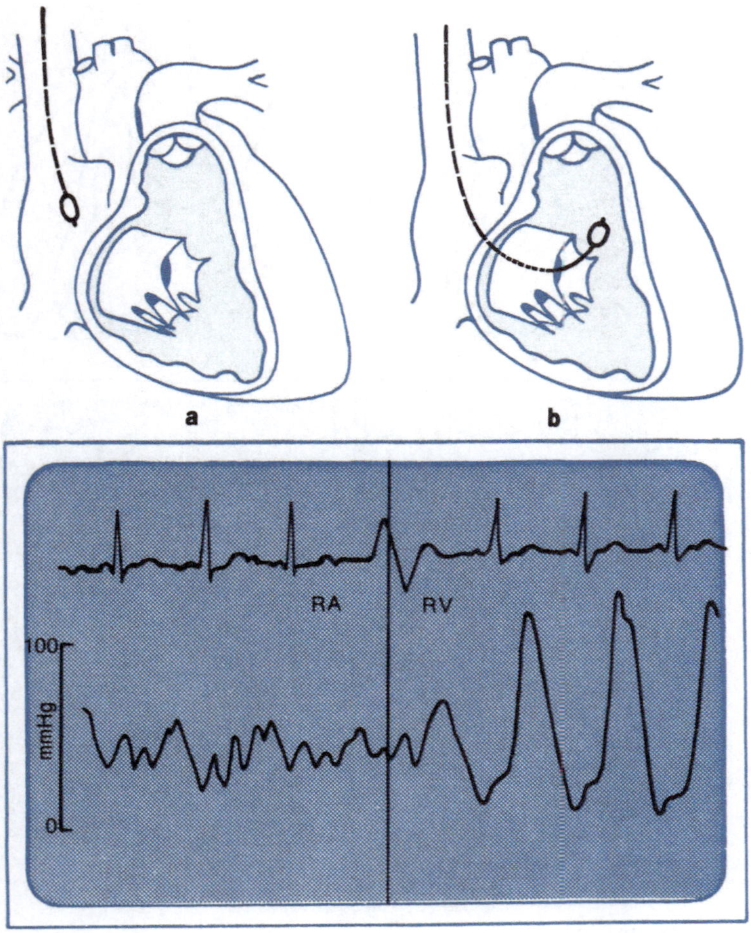

Fig. 18 - Pressure tracing during Swan-Ganz catheter insertion
a) Catheter tip positionned in right atrium (RA)
b) Catheter tip positionned in right ventricle (RV)

the balloon fully. Advance the catheter through the tricuspid valve into the right ventricle (RV). Catheter tip entry into the RV is verified by a rapid change in pressure tracing on the CRT (Fig.18b).

Once this is confirmed, advance the catheter further to the pulmonary artery through the pulmonic valve. The tracing on the screen should show a change, with elevation of its diastolic pressure (Fig. 19).

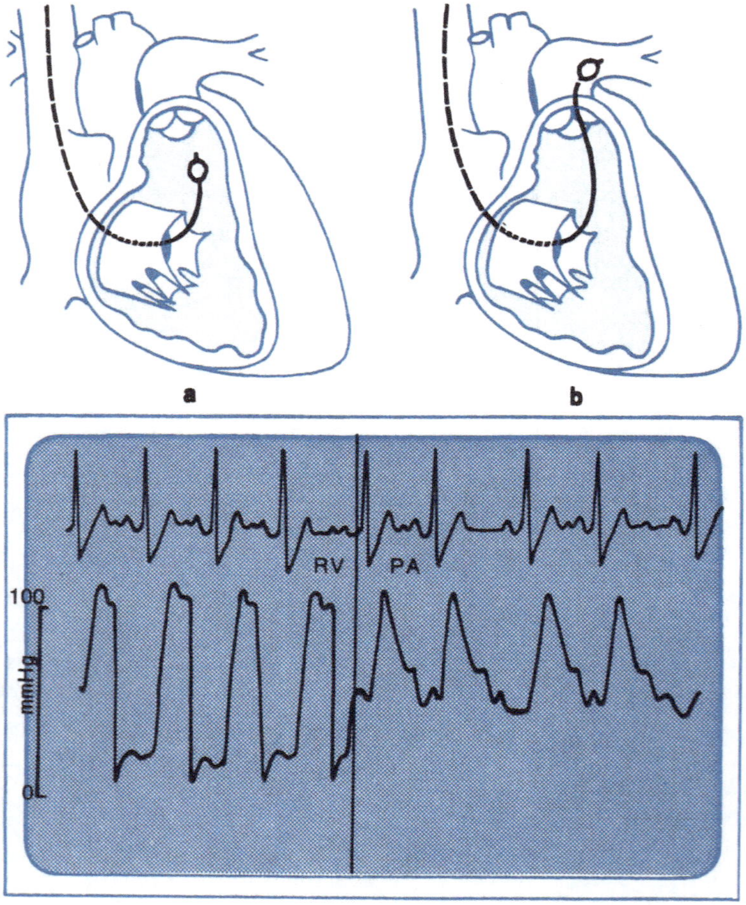

Fig. 19 - Pressure tracing during Swan-Gang catheter insertion
a) Catheter tip positionned in right ventricle (RV)
b) Catheter tip positionned in pulmonary artery (PA)

If this tracing is not observed in spite of approx. 15 cm advancement, the catheter may be kinked or coiled in the right ventricle. In this case, withdraw the catheter 15 cm and advance again. Once in the pulmonary artery, the catheter is advanced until resistance is felt. Deflate the balloon completely and *slightly* advance the catheter. The correct PA pressure is displayed when the catheter is in a stationary position with the balloon deflated.

To obtain pulmonary capillary wedge pressure (PCWP) which is also called pulmonary artery wedge pressure (PAWP), inflate the balloon until the tracing on the CRT changes to a reduced amplitude waveform which is characteristic for PCWP (Fig. 20).

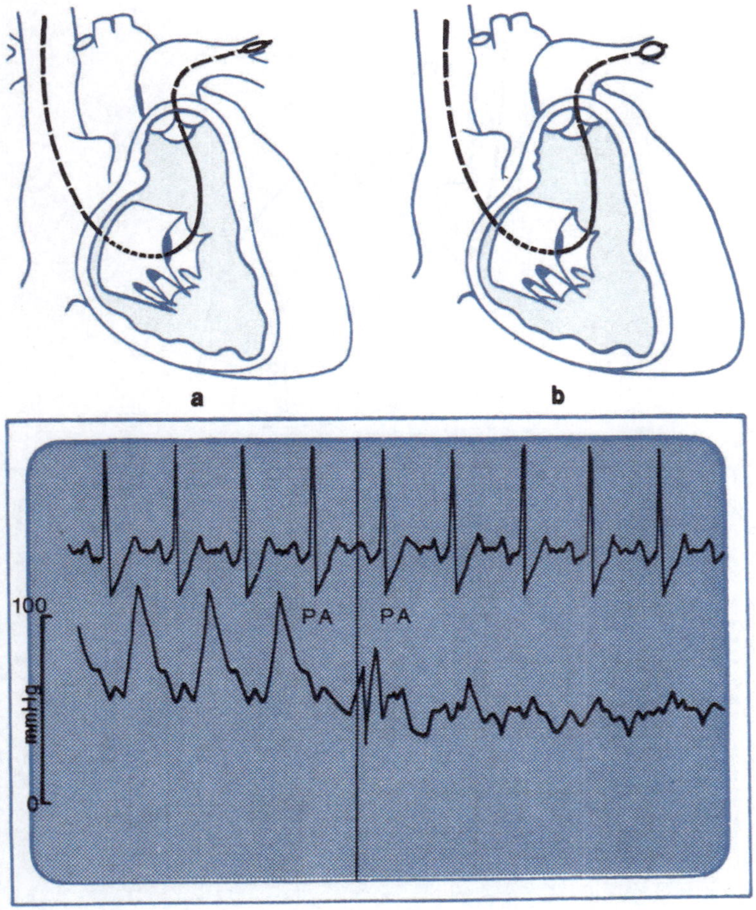

Fig. 20 - Pressure tracing during Swan-Ganz catheter insertion
a) Pulmonary artery(PA), balloon deflated
b) Pulmonary artery (PA), balloon inflated

Inflate the balloon only enough to change the waveform and only for a short time. Take a mean PCWP reading and deflate the balloon. Suture and/or tape the catheter securely in place and apply a sterile dressing to the site of insertion.

11.3. Right atrial (RA) pressure

During a single insertion of a Swan-Ganz catheter there are several additional measurements which may be accomplished at the same time. For example: right atrial pressure. Normal mean RA pressure is 1 to 5 mmHg. Elevation of this pressure may indicate right heart failure, tricuspid stenosis or regurgitation, constrictive pericarditis, pulmonary hypertension, volume overload, and ultimately left ventricular failure. The normal RA tracing has three positive waves for each cardiac cycle (Fig. 21).

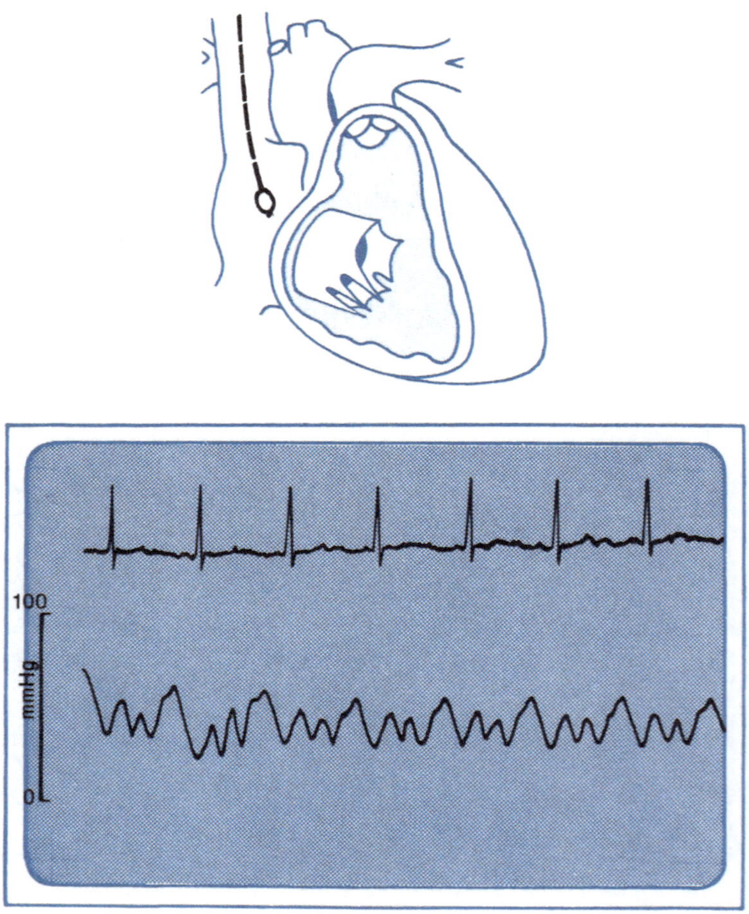

Fig. 21 • Typical RA waveform

The a-wave indicates atrial systole, the descent (x) following the a-wave represents the decline in pressure following atrial systole. The subsequent c-wave represents the movement of the tricuspid valve toward the atrium during valve closure. The peak of the c-wave occurs with the opening of the pulmonary valve. The v-wave represents ventricular systole and its descent (y) represents opening of the tricuspid valve allowing the blood to flow into the right ventricle.

11.4. Right ventricular (RV) pressure

Another clinically significant by product of a Swan-Ganz catheter insertion is RV Pressure. The normal RV systolic pressure is 20 to 30 mmHg. The end-diastolic RV pressure normally is less than 5 mmHg. Abnormal elevation of either or both may be seen with pulmonary hypertension, pulmonary valvular stenosis, right heart failure, constrictive pericarditis, chronic congestive heart failure, ventricular spetal defect etc. The typical normal RV tracing (Fig. 22) will show several phases. During systole, the

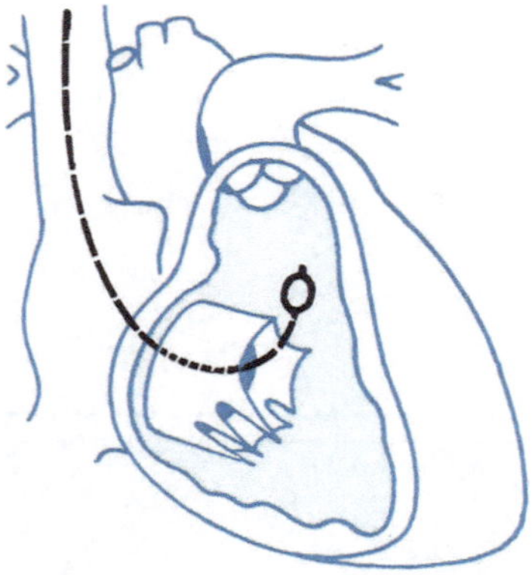

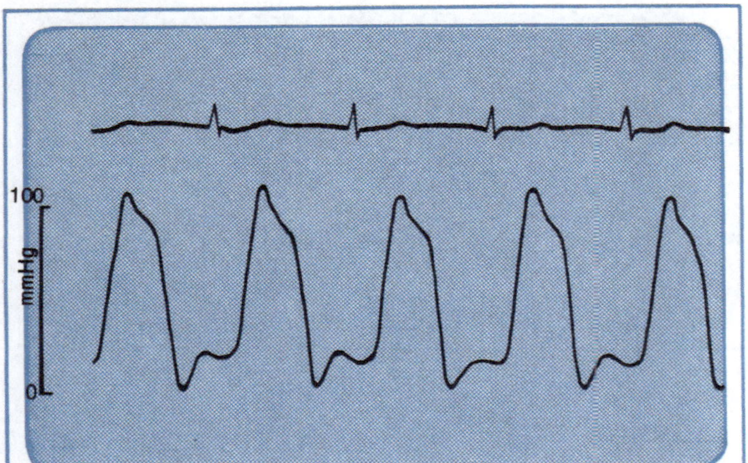

Fig. 22 - Typical RV waveform

first phase occurs after the tricuspid valve closes but before the pulmonary valve opens (isometric contraction). This rapid increase in blood pressure contained in a closed ventricle finally exceeds the PA pressure and opens the pulmonary valve. The ejection phase ensues and lasts until the pulmonary valve closes. Diastole occurs when the heart muscle relaxes. During this phase, the pulmonary valve closes and the tricuspid valve opens to allow the blood to fill the ventricle(s). The filling then continues but at a slower rate until the next systole.

11.5. Pulmonary artery (PA) pressure

In a sense, the pulmonary artery pressure tracings (Fig. 23) are similar to aortic

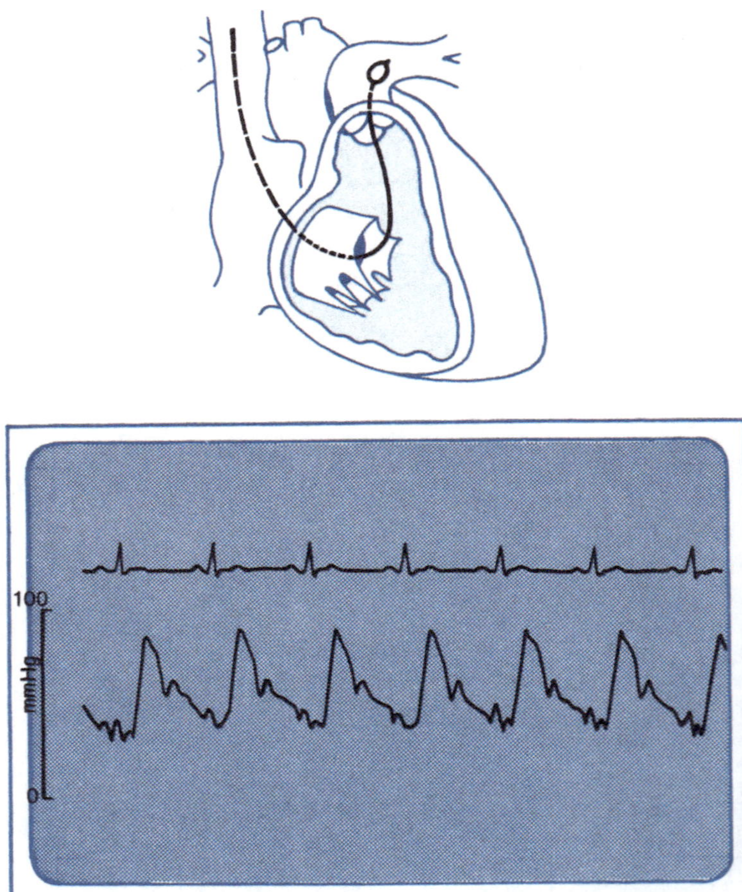

Fig. 23 - Typical PA waveform

pressure. They show a steep rise during RV contraction and ejection flollowing opening of the pulmonary valve. The gradual decrease in pressure follows while blood is ejected from the ventricle until closure of the pulmonary valve. This closure is marked by a dichrotic notch on the PA tracing. Further decline in pressure continues until the minimum end diastolic pressure is reached to be followed immediately by the next systole.

Normal systolic PA pressure is 20 to 30 mmHg; diastolic should be less than 10 mmHg and mean PA pressure lies somewhere in between. Elevated PA pressures may indicate: increased pulmonary blood flow (as in septal defects), increased pulmonary vascular impedance (as in pulmonary hypertension and mitral stenosis) or LV failure from any cause.

11.6. Pulmonary capillary wedge pressure (PCWP)

It is also referred to as pulmonary artery wedge pressure (PAWP). Its waveform (Fig. 24) is similar to LA Pressure. It is also similar to RA tracings in the sense that

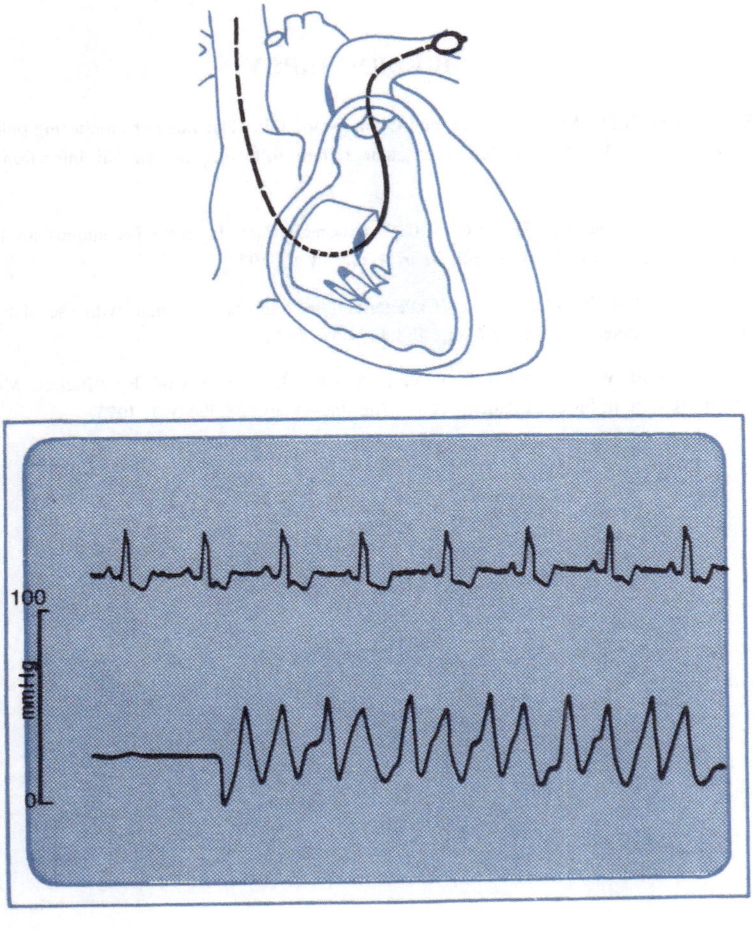

Fig. 24 • Typical PCWP waveform

there are a, c, v, waves and x, y descents.The a-wave occurs during left atrial systole and is usually in the form of a distinct peak in the PCWP tracing. It usually immediately follows the P-wave on ECG tracing. In atrial fibrillation the a-ware disappears. The c-wave indicates the closure of mitral and tricuspid valves at the initiation of ventricular systole. It is the smallest feature on the PCWP tracing and often completely invisible. The v-wave represents the bulging of mitral valve back into the atrium during ventricular systole. It corresponds in timing to the T-wave on the ECG trace. If the valve is incompetent, the v-wave is abnormally high because blood regurgitates back to the left atrium during ventricular systole. In a normal situation the mean PCWP should be nearly the same as the PA diastolic pressure. This means that when the balloon is inflated there should be a noticeable fall in pressure. The normal mean PCWP Pressure averages 4 to 12 mmHg. The difference between maximum and minimum of the a and v-waves is usually small — on the order of 5 mmHg. The elevated PCWP *means* pressure may indicate left ventricular failure, mitral stenosis or mitral insufficiency of any cause.

BIBLIOGRAPHY

1. RUTHERFORD, B.D., McCann, W.D. and O'Donovan, T.P.: The value of monitoring pulmonary artery pressure for early detection of left ventricular failure following myocardial infarction. Circulation, 43:655-665, 1971.

2. RACKLEY, Ch.E. and RUSSEL JR., R.O.: "Coronary Care: Invasive Techniques for Hemodynamic Measurements" published by *American Heart Assoc., N.Y.*, 1973.

3. SWAN, J.H.C., GANZ, W., ET.al.; "Catheterization of the heart in man with use of a flow-directed balloon-tipped catheter". *N.Engl.J.Med.*, 283:447-451, 1970.

4. LAPPAS, D., Lell, W.A. Gabel. J.C., CIVETTA, J.M., LOWENSTEIN, E.: "Indirect Measurement of Left Atrial Pressure in Surgical Patients etc.". Anesthesiology, 38:394-397, 1973.

PROBLEMS AND ERRORS WITH SWAN-GANZ CATHETERS

Problem	*Cause*	*Prevention*	*Remedy*
Damped tracing.	Partial clotting at catheter tip. Tip impacting against vessel wall.	Use continuous flush. Occasionally flush with large volume after blood withdrawal. Carefully advance catheter.	Aspirate blood from catheter then flush with heparinized fluid. Reposition catheter.
Damped tracing with no improvement after flushing.	Forward migration of catheter or air bubble in transducer.	Check catheter position with X-ray. Carefully assemble and flush pressure tubing and transducer.	Pull back catheter, check position with X-ray. Flush system.
Abnormally low or negative pressure.	Transducer level incorrect. Loose connection. Incorrect zero and calibration on monitor.	Maintain or return patient to same position for each reading. Assemble system carefully. Zero and calibrate properly.	Remeasure transducer level, reposition. Check tubing connections. Check zero and calibration on monitor.
Ventricular extrasystoles.	Looping of excess catheter in RV. Migration of tip from PA to RV.	Carefully advance and suture catheter at insertion.	Reposition catheter.
Pulmonary hemorrhage or infarction.	Prolonged wedging of catheter. Balloon overinflation.	Leave balloon deflated between measurements. Do not forcefully flush when in wedge position.	Remove catheter.
Painful inflammed insertion site.	Thrombophlebitis due to irritation and/or infection.	Use sterile technique. Wet catheter thoroughly during insertion. Insert smoothly. Change dressings, stopcock and tubing daily.	Apply warm compress. Elevate arm. Medicate pain.
Inappropriate waveform.	Altered catheter tip location. Movement of tip against wall.	Suture catheter at insertion. Hard to avoid.	Check position on X-ray and reposition catheter.
No pressure readout.	Transducer stopcock not open to catheter. Monitor controls in wrong position.	Follow step-by-step procedure for assembly, zero, calibration and flushing of monitoring system.	Check stopcocks. Check monitor.

Table III

XII - DIRECT PRESSURE MONITORING IN INFANTS

The early diagnosis and management of abnormal blood pressure in enfants is as important or even more essential than that in the adult patient. It is in the first 48 hours of a newborn life that the cardiovascular system is the most unstable and this is when blood pressure determination and correction can significantly reduce the infant morbidity and mortality. It may effectively detect signs of infant respiratory distress and persistet fetal circulation. It can help to diagnose the early symptoms and to manage impending cardiogenic shock due to congenital defects, thereby literally saving the life of a newborn. Direct blood pressure monitoring of infants has not yet reached widespread routine application largely due to its apparent complexity and the high degree of skill required of medical personnel. The purpose of this Chapter is to explain the issues involved in order to make their understanding easier and thereby overcome resistance to routine blood pressure monitoring.

12.1. Preparation of materials

While the assembly of the pressure monitoring system, i.e. catheter, stopcocks, tubing, flush devices, fluid sources and the transducer are essentially the same as in adult monitoring (see Chapter 8) special care is required for flushing procedure. To avoid the clot formation the catheters should be continuously flushed. It is possible to use an Intraflo device with a slow infusion rate of 3 ml/hr, but better yet is to use of calibrated (motorized) infusion pumps for accurate control of the flush fluid flow. This is because in infants the fluid intake must often be limited to very small volumes (not to exceed 25 ml/day).

12.2. Monitoring and insertion sites

As in adult monitoring, the pressures of interest in infants include: systemic arterial, central venous, right heart, pulmonary artery and pulmonary capillary wedge. Due to the much smaller size of vessels in these tiny patients, the insertion techniques and sites differ slightly from those used in adults.

For monitoring systemic arterial pressure in infants less than 72 hours old, the umbilical artery is the most common insertion site. Other but less commonly used arterial insertion sites are brachial, axillary, radial and temporal arteries. Use of femoral arteries should be avoided because of the possibility of vascular complications.

For measurements of venous, right heart and pulmonary artery pressures, the balloon-tip (Swan-Ganz) catheter is inserted into one of the large veins, e.g. femoral or axillary. Use of the balloon-tip catheter is especially advantageous in infants with complex congenital heart defects. The catheter floating downstream with the blood can easily reach those vessels or chambers of the heart which may be difficult to access by other means. It is a good practice to use *carbon dioxide* instead of air to inflate the balloon when monitoring children with right-to-left shunts. This is to avoid the risk of systemic air emboli in case of accidental balloon rupture. When air is released during rupture it will not dissolve in blood and may cause partial embolic damage to affected organs. The carbon dioxide on the other hand, is blood-soluble and will seldom cause serious side effects.

12.3. Insertion techniques

After assembling the monitoring system and properly flushing, zeroing and calibrating, everything is ready for catheter insertion.

For umbilical artery monitoring the umbilical stump is prepared with Betadine or iodine and alcohol. The incision is made on the artery under sterile conditions. The Intracath cannula is passed into the artery far enough to ensure stability. The largest bore catheter which the artery will accommodate should be lubricated with sterile glycerine and pushed into the artery. Caution should be exercised not to cause arterial spasm or vessel perforation. This is one of the reasons for the use of softer catheters than in adults. (Fig. 25).

For venous insertion, a standard venous cutdown technique is used as the veins are usually too small to accommodate the guide needle used for adults. The larger vein (femoral or axillary) must be catheterized under sterile conditions, of course.

12.4. Complications and specific features

The complications which may ensue following umbilical artery catheterization include: thrombosis, embolization, hemorrhage and infection. It has been reported that renal artery thrombosis occurs in less than 5% of the catheterized infants. The infants should be observed carefully and frequently for signs of hypertension (indicative of renal artery thrombosis) or cyanosis of lower torso and extremities.

The reduce the incidence of complications following arterial catheterization the catheter tip should be advanced to the level of the aortic bifurcation, and blood pressure should be monitored during and *following* the period of catheterization.

For venous catheterization, all the complications of adult monitoring described in Chapter 9 are applicable to infants. Arrhythmias and temporary hypotension may occur during passage or the catheter through the heart chambers.

12.5. Summary

When indicated, the monitoring of blood pressure in infants is as feasible as in adults. The differences in size of catheterized vessels, insertion techniques and special precautions are easy to adjust to. The basic principles and diagnostic benefits from pressure monitoring of infants are the same as in adult patients.

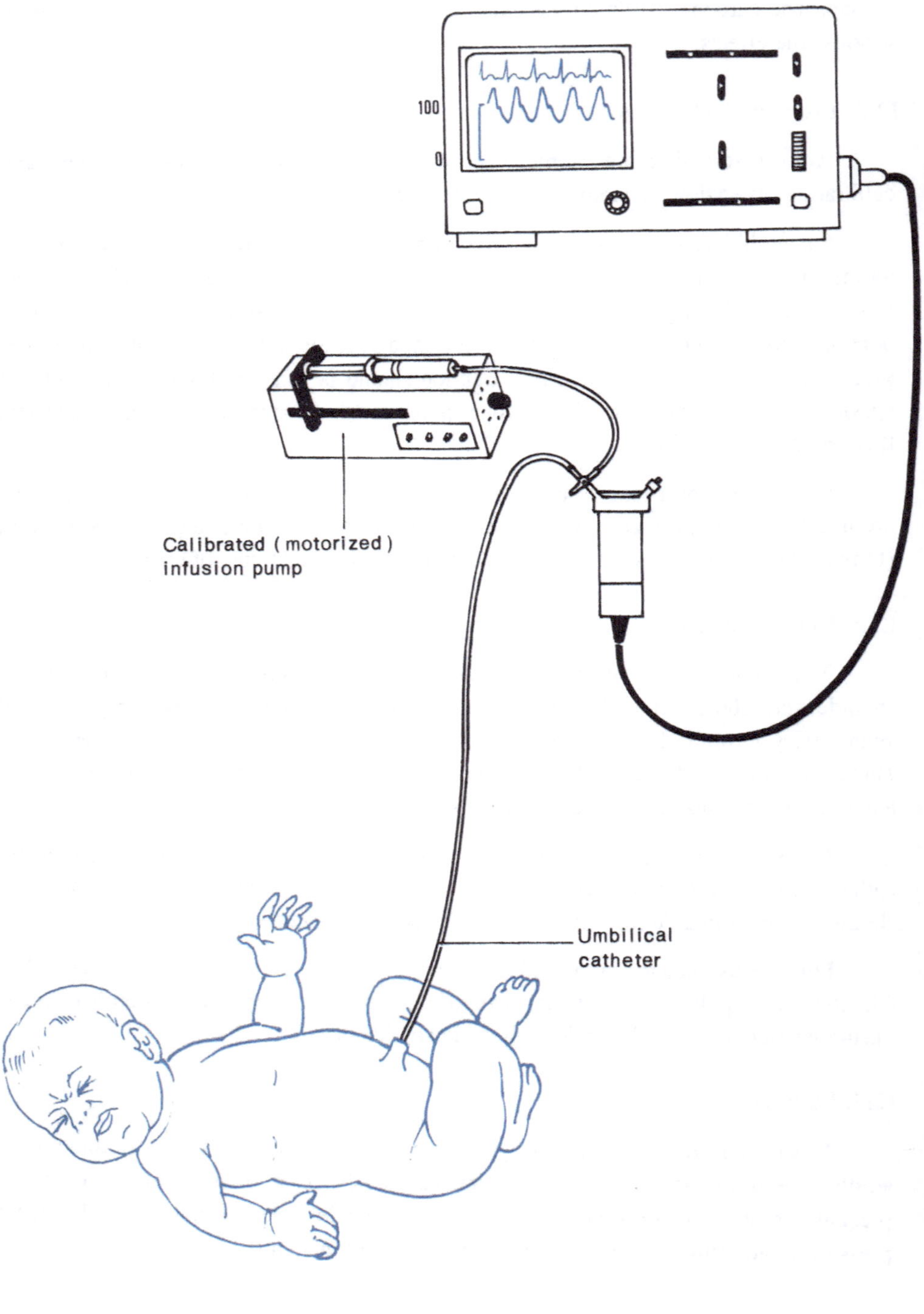

Fig. 25 - Direct umbilical artery pressure monitoring in infants

XIII - CLINICAL ASPECTS AND DISCUSSION OF HEMODYNAMIC MONITORING

13.1. Long-term intravascular monitoring

Intravascular pressures, including central venous, right atrial, pulmonary arterial (including PAWP), and systemic arterial pressure can be continuously monitored for long periods of time in patients with cardiovascular problems. This becomes especially valuable for patients with acute myocardial infarction and also in cardiac postoperative cases. The hard-copy record of these pressure tracings or just measurements of their values can and should be made every thirty minutes and entered in the patient's progress chart. With a Swan-Ganz catheter in a pulmonary artery the balloon should not be left inflated and the return of a pulmonary arterial tracing should be ascertained after each balloon deflation.

13.2. Pressure monitoring in myocardial infarction

Patients with uncomplicated myocardial infarction (MI), characterized by the absence of arrhytmias and heart failure, generally have more or less normal cardiac pressures. Measurements of pressure indicate RA pressure 5±2 mm, pulmonary artery end-diastolic pressure of 11±4 mmHg and PA mean pressure of 15±5 mmHg. In these patients the left ventricular end diastolic pressure, measured as PCWP, was found to be 16±9 mmHg. (Rackley & Russell[1]).

Patients with acute MI resulting in *mild* congestive heard failure characterized by basal rales and ventricular gallop have RA pressure 8±4 mmHg, PA end-diastolic pressure of 21±10 mmHg and mean PA pressure of 27±7 mmHg (Wolk, et.al[2]). Their PCWP which corresponded to left ventricular end-diastolic pressure (LVEDP) was 25±7 mmHg.

In *severe* congestive heart failure and advanced pulmonary edema, consistent pressure measurements are difficult to obtain as the patients often cannot lie in the supine position. The reported findings suggest that an increase of pulmonary artery end-diastolic pressure (PAEDP) above 25 mmHg and LVEDP above 25 mmHg are the criteria for severe heart failure classification.

Patients in severe cardiogenic *shock* with clinical evidence of reduced organ perfusion, arterial systolic pressure below 90 mmHg, arrhythmia and severe pain have been studied and the PAEDP was found at 25±13 mmHg, LVEDP at 24±12 mmHg.

As studied by Rutherford[3], the clinical course in patients with acute MI and mean PA pressure less than 20 mmHg, was stable with a favorable prognosis for survival. On the other hand patients with mean PA pressure above 20 mmHg have higher incidences of arrhythmia, hemodynamic complications and death during the immediate post-infarction period.

13.3. Respiratory effects on RA and PA pressures

Both PA and RA pressure will fluctuate as the intrathoracic and intrapulmonic pressures change in the course of respiration. At the resting end expiratory level, the intrapulmonic pressure is atmospheric, i.e., 0 mmHg in reference to air (and blood pressure zero reference). During inspiration it becomes negative (– 2 to – 3 mmHg) in order to inhale air to the lungs. These changes are reflected in pressure changes in the intrathoracic space which are even greater than intrapulmonary pressure and range from – 5 to – 8 mmHg. As the heart and connecting vessels are exposed to this intrathoracic pressure it superimposes itself on whatever pressure is measured in the blood stream. The result is oscillatory pattern of all pressures, including RA and PA visible on the monitor tracing (Fig. 26).

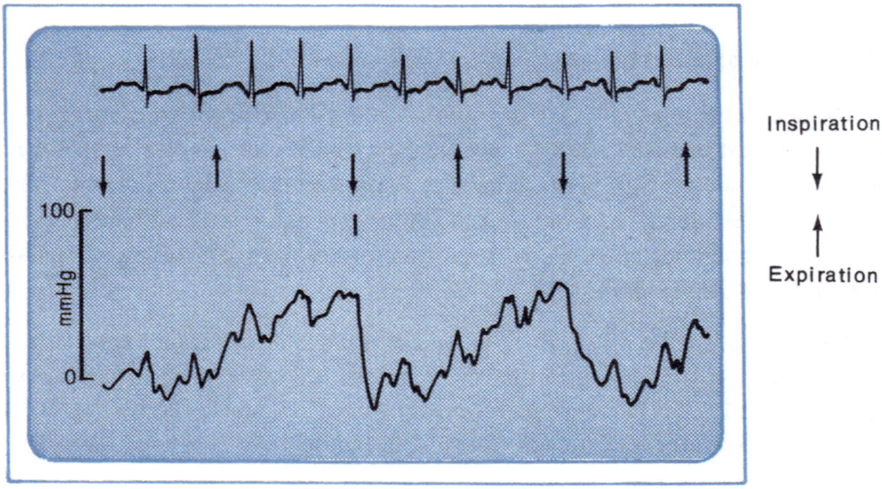

Fig. 26 - Respiration affecting the RA pressure tracing
(time-base 12.5mm/ sec)

The frequency of slow oscillations on the tracing corresponds to the respiratory rhythm. For clinical determinations, the pressure values should be measured during the *expiratory* phase, preferably just before the onset of the pronounced and rapid inspiratory phase fall in pressure.

13.4. PA pressure in mitral insufficiency

It is assumed that for all practical purpose the value of PAEDP (which in turn is virtually equal to mean PCWP) reflects accurately LA and in consequence LVEDP. In patients with mitral stenosis there is a severe disparity between these values which varies according to the severity of the condition. This is due to obstruction between the atrium and ventricle; the pressures do not have time to equilibrate during the end-diastolic filling phase. Thus conclusions based on an elevated PAEDP may be totally meaningless in these cases and lead to erroneous therapeutic strategy. Therefore it is essential to establish that there is no mitral disease before interpreting the results obtained in the pulmonary artery and pulmonary capillary wedge position.

BIBLIOGRAPHY

1. RACKLEY, C.E. AND RUSSELL, R.O.: "Coronary Care: Invasive techniques for hemodynamic measurements", *published by American Heart Assoc., N.Y.*, 1973.

2. WOLK, M.J., SCHEIDT, S., KILIP, T.: "Heart failure complicating acute myocardial infarction", *Circulation*, **45:1125,** 1972.

3. RUTHERFORD, B.D., McCANN, W.D., O'DONOVAN, R.O.Jr: "The value of monitoring PA pressure for early detection of left ventricular failure following myocardial infarction", *Circulation*, **43:655,** 1971.

XIV - DIRECT INTRACRANIAL PRESSURE MONITORING

The delicate structures of the brain and spinal cord are surrounded by the protective barrier of the cerebrospinal (CSF) fluid. The CSF fills the intracranial and spinal cavities. The continuous measurement of cerebrospinal fluid pressure provides information for patient management. This concerns patients with brain edema, obstructed CSF channels, cerebral space occupying lesions, and intracranial hypertension. The above conditions usually result in *elevation* of CSF pressure.

Intracranial CSF pressure also is one of the factors associated with cerebral blood perfusion. The CSF pressure is approximately the same as the pressure in cerebral veins and it tends to parallel any changes in their pressure. Studies on traumatic head injuries suggest that some patients demonstrate brain ischemia and impaired neurological function associated with rise of CSF pressure to 20-25 mmHg. The mean normal value of CSF pressure is 5-7 mmHg. It is also apparent in head injuries that the cause of increased CSF pressure is more important than elevation of pressure in itself.

14.1. Insertion sites

The three sites commonly used for intracranial pressure monitoring are:

— intraventricular

— subdural or subarachnoid

— epidural

For intraventricular monitoring the tip of a fluid-filled catheter is placed in a frontal horn of the lateral ventricle.Subdural or subarachnoid technique uses shallow penetration of the dura matter by a mini-transducer or a hollow screw connected to a pressure transducer via fluid-filled tubing.

Both of the above methods, although commonly used today, entail invasion of brain space beyond the dura surface. This carries the risk of infection, brain trauma or loss of CSF. The method of choice is the use of minitransducers placed directly over the dura (epidural) just below the inner surface of the skull. The main problem, at present, is imperfect transducer technology which is responsible for less widespread use of the epidural method.

14.2. Insertion techniques

For intraventricular catheterization, a sterile burr hole is drilled in the frontal region of the skull and approximately 7 cm length of ventricular catheter is introduced. The catheter tip should reach the frontal horn of the lateral ventricle, which is confirmed by a slow rise in the pressure on the monitor. (Fig. 27)

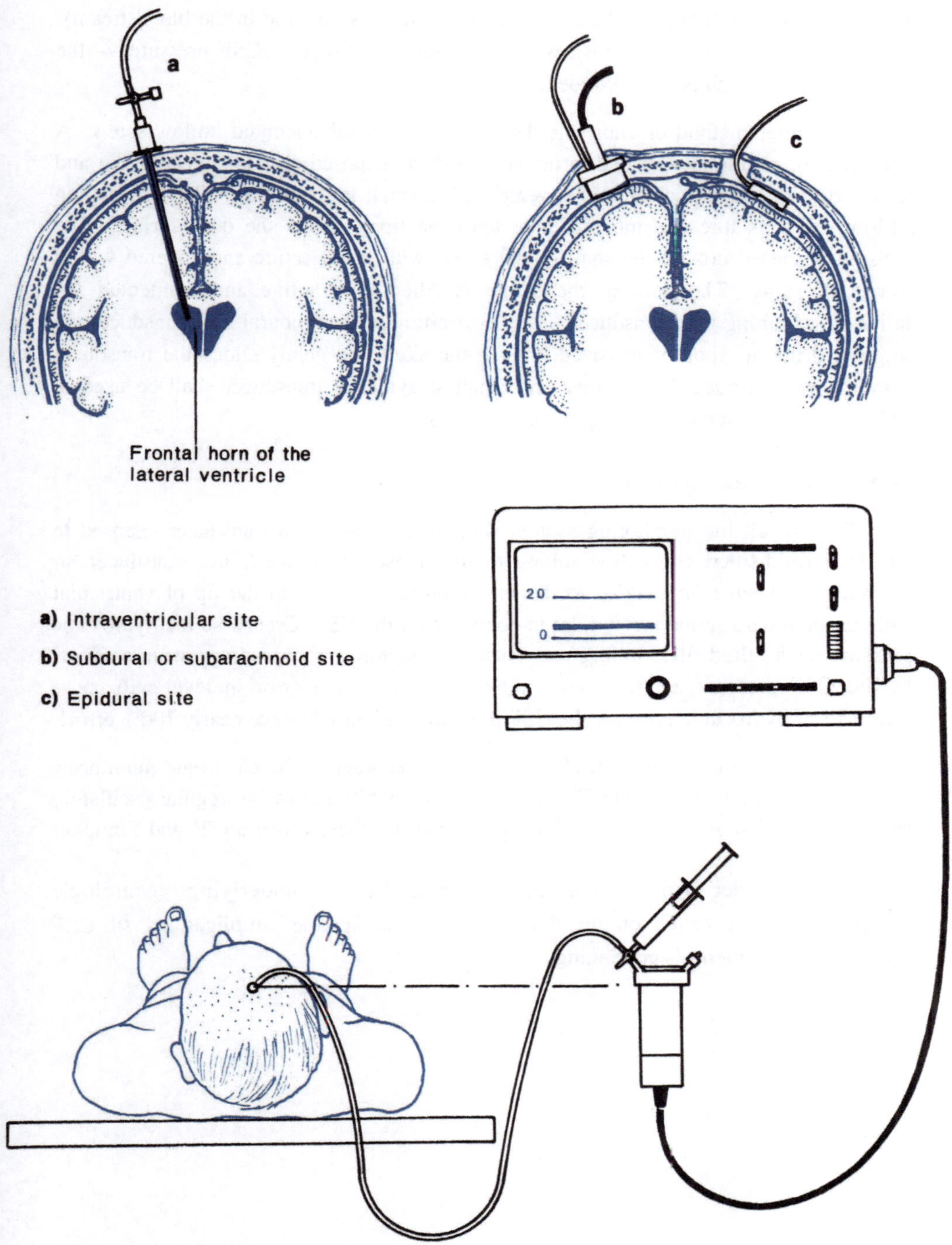

Fig. 27 - Direct intracranial pressure monitoring

The continuous *flush* devices *must not be used* in connection with the catheter-transducer tubing as there is no clotting (as was the case in the bloodstream). Furthermore, the continuous flush would contribute to a rise in CSF pressure — the very condition which is to be avoided.

The other method of choice is the insertion of a subarachnoid hollow screw. A 1/4'' (ca. 6 mm) hole is drilled in the skull and the exposed dura is delicately cut and removed to expose the arachnoid covered with a small layer of CSF. The self-tapping hollow screw is threaded into the hole until the tip is below the dura surface. The incision is closed around the shaft of the screw with a silk suture and covered with a sterile dressing. The hole in the screw is filled with saline and connected via saline-filled tubing to a transducer. For the insertion of the epidural minitransducer the surgeon drills an appropriate sized hole in the skull and gently slides the transducer over the dura surface. The flattest and smallest available transducer shall be used in order to avoid erroneously high pressure readings.

14.3. Pressure measurements

First of all the monitoring system should be zeroed with transducer exposed to air. If a fluid-filled connection tubing to the transducer is used, the transducer air reference port *must be levelled* to the measurement site, i.e. to the tip of ventricular catheter or subarachnoid screw inlet in contact with the CSF. Otherwise the hydrostatic pressure in the fluid-filled tubing will cause very significant errors in pressure readouts as the CSF pressure are low. For example, as the 7 cm error in level will cause 5 mmHg of hydrostatic pressure the CSF pressure readout will have nearly 100% error!

An addition of a slow speed (ca. 5 cm/hr) recorder to the electronic monitoring system is essential because the CSF pressure often exhibits slow but regular oscillatory pattern, so-called A or B waves. The cycle times for these waves are 20 and 5 minutes respectively.

The character of these waves may be indicative of underlying neurologic symptoms. The research on the diagnostic and therapeutic implications of CSF pressure measurements is continuing.

XV - DIRECT AMNIOTIC FLUID PRESSURE MONITORING

During labor the uterine contractions exert pressure on the fetus. This may stress the fetal circulatory system and cause a slowing of fetal heart rate immediately following the uterine contraction. This slowing of the heart rate provides a gross indication of severe stress and impairment of circulation in the fetus. If such stress is forceful and persistent over a long time it may result in brain ischemia and consequent partial damage. Hence the need arise for knowledge of the forces acting over the fetus in order to undertake appropriate intervention when prolonged increase in pressure produces a significant drop in fetal heart rate. These pressures can be measured indirectly by an external abdominal force transducer (so-called tocograph). The direct pressure is a method of choice as it is more reliable.

15.1. Intrauterine pressure monitoring

A similar setup is used as for other pressure measurements. There is *no need* for a continuous flush system. The transducer reference port should be leveled to the anatomic level of symphysis pubis of the woman in labor. Prior to monitoring, a large bore, stiff catheter should be filled with saline and connected to a transducer via a flexible extension tubing. The catheter tip is then introduced through the dilated cervix following the rupture of membranes and the monitoring is carried out. (fig. 28).

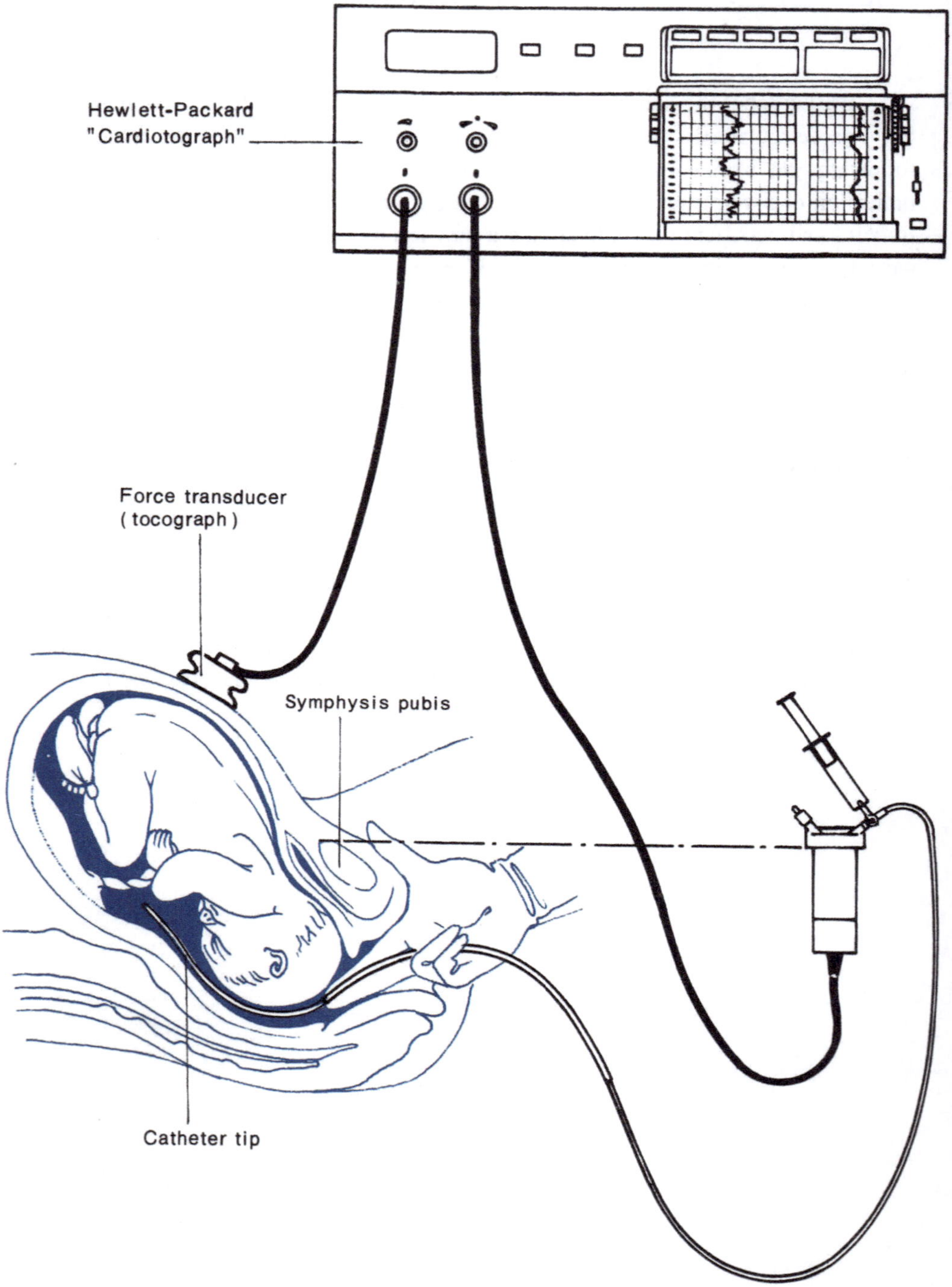

Fig. 28 - Direct amniotic fluid pressure monitoring

SUBJECT INDEX

TABLE OF PLATES

3779 - Imprimerie Bayeusaine
6, rue Royale, 14401 Bayeux
N° dépôt légal 4198 - 4e trimestre 1980

GPSR Compliance

The European Union's (EU) General Product Safety Regulation (GPSR) is a set of rules that requires consumer products to be safe and our obligations to ensure this.

If you have any concerns about our products, you can contact us on ProductSafety@springernature.com

In case Publisher is established outside the EU, the EU authorized representative is:

Springer Nature Customer Service Center GmbH
Europaplatz 3
69115 Heidelberg, Germany

Batch number: 10620854

Printed by Printforce, the Netherlands